THE CARING SERVICES

Bill Clark
MA(Hons) DSW CQSW DPA

Churchill Livingstone

EDINBURGH LONDON MADRID MELBOURNE NEW YORK AND TOKYO 1993

CHURCHILL LIVINGSTONE
Medical Division of Longman Group UK Limited

Distributed in the United States of America by Churchill Livingstone Inc., 650 Avenue of the Americas, New York, NY 10011, and by associated companies, branches and representatives throughout the world.

First published 1993

ISBN 0-443-04527-5

British Library Cataloguing In Publication Data
A catalogue record for this book is available from the British Library.

Library of Congress Cataloging in Publication Data
A catalog record for this book is available from the Library of Congress.

For Churchill Livingstone

Publisher: Mary Law
Project Manager: Ellen Green
Editor: Valerie Bain
Production Controller: Mark Sanderson
Design: Design Resources Unit
Sales Promotion Executive: Hilary Brown

Produced by Longman Singapore Publishers Pte Ltd
Printed in Singapore

The
publisher's
policy is to use
**paper manufactured
from sustainable forests**

Contents

To the reader

Here are some questions which may occur to you before you start to read this book

Who is this book for?

Anyone involved in caring. It has been designed with you – the reader – in mind. We've tried to make it look and feel friendly and attractive.

Do I need to enrol in a course to use this book?

*Certainly not, although you may find that it is used by many Caring courses. The books in the **Skills for Caring** series are for anyone involved in caring. You can use it on your own, at your workplace as part of an assessment programme if you're in employment, or as part of a more formal training programme at a college or other institution.*

Where can I read this book?

Anywhere you like. You can read it in 'snatches', if this is more convenient for you, or you can interrupt your reading to do some of the exercises. It may help you to write on it, if it's your own copy. As you will see, the book has been designed to be used in a very flexible way.

Are there any special features that I should be aware of before starting to read this book?

You'll find it a great help to know the following:

Definitions:
*Sometimes a key word might be unfamiliar to some readers, or we might want to be sure that the **precise** meaning is clear. We've tried to pick out such words and give their meaning at the place where the word is first mentioned. The word and its definition have been set off in a box.*

Examples:
There's no substitute for a good example to make a point or convey a message. We've included as many examples as possible and have set these off from the main text with boxes, so that you can skip them if you like, or locate them again if you found them particularly helpful.

Exercises:
*These have been set off from the text in a different colour. The exercises can extend your knowledge considerably and reinforce what you've read in the main text. You can do the exercises on your own, with a group, or under the direction of a tutor. Or you can choose **not** to do them at all, or to do them later, after you've read and absorbed the text. The choice is yours. Remember: This is **your** book – enjoy it!*

Introduction

■ *Working in the caring services can provide a rewarding and meaningful career. Individuals, families, groups and communities often benefit greatly from the commitment and talents of care workers and the resources provided by the caring services. But caring is not a simple task. Anyone involved in care or caring has to face up to complexity, conflicts and contradictions in his or her daily work. This book has been written to help all people who are, or wish to be, care workers make sense of their task in the context of the health and welfare services in the United Kingdom.*

CARE AND CARING

There will always be apparent contradictions about care and caring. Continuity and consistency in caring are often considered to be the basis of good care yet the main health and welfare agencies have spent the last few years caught up in constant change and reorganisation in response to central government policy initiatives.

The most intimate acts of personal care are often undertaken by relative strangers. The majority of care workers are employed by massive state agencies set up to deal with large-scale social problems. But the work of these carers and service providers often involves small-scale human encounters between people. These caring exchanges work best when people are sensitive to each other's feelings, but the organisational pressures of working in big institutions like hospitals, or bureaucracies such as the social services, sometimes make it difficult to take the time to be sensitive.

The big providers of health and social care often employ professional groups of staff like nurses, social workers and doctors. At times professional and organisational approaches to care can inhibit sensitivity to people, and emotional involvement with them, because agency systems, procedures and rules have to be followed.

A significant number of the people who most need care and protection don't want it; the need to receive care is often associated with personal rejection or failure.

All aspects of care and the caring services suggest that the issues surrounding them are complex.

1

What is caring?

■ Although 'caring' for people has universal appeal as a 'good' thing there is some difficulty in defining what it is all about. 'Caring' can mean many things to many people. It is a skilled business (whether it's done by people who are paid or not for doing it), and involves 3 elements, all of which have to be put together to make it work.

See Exercise 1.

● ●

EXERCISE 1

Think about yourself in a caring role. This might be in your present job (care worker) or when you've cared for someone who's a relative or a friend (informal carer), or what you imagine it might be like to be a care worker (such as a home help or a worker in a residential home for children).

• As a care worker, write down some of the things you have to *know, feel and do* to be a good carer. Write down your ideas under the headings:

• Knowing • Feeling • Doing

● ●

There are no simple answers to Exercise 1. It can be difficult to decide how to describe certain qualities of caring. Your list probably included some things that might have gone in any of the columns. This is because caring is about a state of mind as well as activity.

Look at the following examples of caring and decide for yourself which aspect of caring is most important to the task.

• **To be lifted off a toilet seat roughly by someone who is angry with you (and shows it) is probably an assault rather than caring.**
• **To have your shopping bought for you and**

find all the wrong things in the bag is careless caring.
• **To be told to fill in a form for a social security benefit for which you are not entitled is thoughtless caring.**
• **To be blind and be guided (by a kind person) into a closed door, because they don't understand guiding technique, is to be on the receiving end of negligence.**
• **To find that a new carer looking after you has no idea how your care was planned or provided in the past is evidence of lazy caring.**

To be careful, or 'full of care', means showing great concern for the other person and for the way duties and tasks are performed. It doesn't really matter what the caring is about. This book and others in the *Skills for Caring Series* try to define competence or 'good caring' for all care workers.

VALUES, PRINCIPLES AND KNOWLEDGE

In several of the examples we asked you to think about there was evidence that the care worker's feelings were not right for the task. The values and principles that care workers carry with them into their work are important elements of good caring. The terms 'values' and 'principles' are used to describe the right feelings and standards that help you judge how to think and behave as a care worker.

Caring also involves applying skills in helping people to do things for themselves, or for them if they are not able to manage by themselves. Skills can be taught and be learned. Sometimes experience provides the best understanding.

The other side of caring involves acquiring information and learning or understanding about people, their lives and the services that might be helpful to them. This book is largely about getting to know the main sources of support and help that should be available for people who need care.

THE CORE OF CARE

So far, we haven't really offered a definition of 'care'. We've laid out some of the features of good care but we need to try and spell out what is at the core of care.

One social work writer (Ainsworth 1985) sees care at the centre of 4 types of positive action (see Figure 1):

- **treating**
- **teaching**
- **nurturing**
- **controlling.**

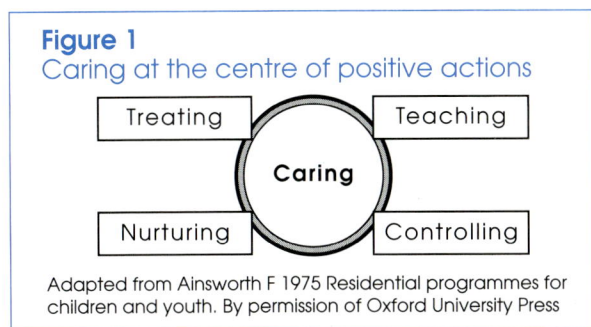

Figure 1
Caring at the centre of positive actions

Treating — Teaching
Caring
Nurturing — Controlling

Adapted from Ainsworth F 1975 Residential programmes for children and youth. By permission of Oxford University Press

This framework seems a good starting point to define care, but our definition needs to take account of the range of roles and activities that care workers often have to undertake. Care workers are:

- **supporters – they get alongside people and help**
- **therapists and counsellors – they actively help people deal with physical and emotional problems**
- **caretakers – they provide basic physical care and protection when this is needed**
- **advisors – they give 'expert' advice when this is requested and appropriate**
- **educators – they pass on skills and knowledge**
- **administrators – they organise themselves and their time and are accountable through recording and other systems for the services they provide**
- **brokers – they link people to other services**
- **coordinators – they make sure that their work fits in with the needs and wishes of people and the planned use of other services and carers**
- **advocates – they push for resources to meet the needs they and their service users identify and they try to influence the way their own organisation and others deliver services.**

In applying all of these skills care workers have to identify and assess people's needs and plan how to meet them. The actual type of care provided by care workers will depend on the needs of their clients, the purpose of their agency and their occupational role, or job, in the setting.

Caring can range from providing continuing intimate physical care to providing information during a one-off interview. Good care, however, in *all* contexts demands that clients are respected as people at *all* times. This means that the carer must always respect the personal choices, privacy, confidentiality, age, gender, sexual identity, cultural, racial and religious identity, and physical and mental condition of the individuals receiving care. Above all, their independence should be encouraged as far as possible. You can read more about this in *Skills for Caring – Clients as Individuals*.

To be effective in their work care workers need to know a great deal about themselves, their own organisation, and what other welfare agencies, like social security, can do to provide support to people.

WHO NEEDS CARE AND GIVES IT?

We know from our discussion about the 'what' of care that care and caring involve many activities, attitudes and organisations. We expect care workers to be concerned, to be responsible, to think about others and to demonstrate their care by using their knowledge, feelings and skills to help others. But is it possible to identify which groups or types of people need care in our society?

Identifying who should receive care and what resources should be made available to them has been a problem faced by every generation of every country or society across the world. In providing answers, each society has to engage in moral, political and economic debate.

WHO NEEDS CARE?

Let's find out which people, groups and communities you think need care and the resources of formal caring services.

Try Exercise 2.

• •

EXERCISE 2

List your 'Top 10' types of people, groups or communities who need care.

• •

There probably isn't a correct answer for Exercise 2 but there might be some ways of assessing the need for care that can help us make the decisions. Let us look at someone else's list of people who need 'caring'. The government's White Paper *Caring for people* (HMSO 1989) and the **Community Care Act 1990**, put forward their idea of the key groups needing community care. The White Paper says:

'Many people need some extra help and support at some stage in their lives, as a result of illness or temporary disability. Some people, as a result of the effects of old age, of mental illness including dementia, of mental handicap (learning disability) or physical disability or sensory impairment, have a continuing need for care on a longer term basis. People with drug and alcohol-related disorders, people with progressive illnesses, such as AIDS or multiple sclerosis, may also need community care at some time.'

The report also notes the specific needs of people from ethnic minority groups and the legislation highlights the needs of children who have 'special needs' as a result of any of these other problems. The needs of carers (that is relatives, friends and neighbours) who pick up the bulk of real responsibility for caring are also mentioned. How close was your list to the government's view?

Community care, in the White Paper, means providing the right level of help and support to people to enable them to lead as full and independent lives as they can – with as much control over their own lives as possible. The 'social care' to be provided ranges from domiciliary support for people in their own homes, with respite care and day care added if required, to more intensive care needs provided through sheltered housing, group living homes and hostels, and finally long-stay hospital care. This range of care has to come from agencies dealing with social care, health and social security payments.

RESPITE: WHEN SOMEONE IS GIVEN CARE BY OTHER PEOPLE THAN THEIR USUAL CARERS, SUCH AS IN A FOSTER HOME OR A WEEKEND BREAK IN A RESIDENTIAL HOME – IT MEANS THE CARE IS 'SHARED' CARE.

There are problems about accepting these definitions of care needs and responses in the community care reforms without question. Definitions of need are sometimes viewed too simply. It seems you either have something wrong with you or you don't – you either need care or you don't. The real world is often more complicated.

There are some key points we can make about needing care. Everybody needs care at some stage in their lives. The need for caring happens throughout each person's life cycle. The need for care arises when we experience dependency. Dependency means that, for whatever reason, we can't look after ourselves or run our own lives. A range of people and services can respond to our dependency.

Each individual's life history will feature significant events or crises.

CRISIS: A TIME WHEN SOMETHING GOES WRONG IN A PERSON'S LIFE OR A TURNING POINT THAT REQUIRES NEW WAYS OF COPING IN LIFE.

There are 2 kinds of crises:

- **Anticipated crises, for example, the dependency of childhood or the frailty of old age.**
- **Unanticipated crises, for example, the disability caused by serious injury, disease or mental breakdown, or the loss created by the death or desertion of a carer or partner.**

The need for care can be temporary or permanent. People caught up in these kinds of experience often need care and support.

Children, as a group, have to be added to our list of vulnerable people who often require caring and support. If the carers of children and young people are affected by the types of life crisis identified then their ability to look after and supervise them can be impaired. Society has evolved systems of care and protection that can be used to help parents and carers fulfil their responsibilities. The same laws and systems can be used, on society's behalf, to take over the role of caring for children and young people if parents and carers cannot meet society's expectations.

One of the factors which complicates health and social care work is that although 2 people might have the same problem they don't always demand, or need, the same services or support. This is partly the result of individual personality and character but it often reflects the social circumstances that confront different people. For this reason, examination of who should receive support and services from caring agencies has to consider the impact of poverty and deprivation.

For over a century, researchers, politicians and professionals working in health and welfare agencies have argued about the causes and effects of poverty and deprivation. Even defining the terms causes debate. One disabled woman defined poverty as 'having too much of the week left at the end of my money' (Casserly and Clark 1978).

When people attempt to live on very low incomes for long periods of time, and live in conditions that are unhealthy or overcrowded, then they suffer from stress. Part of this stress is about not being able to take part in society in the ways other people can. All the groups liable to need care mentioned in this section are more likely to be present in poorer communities where levels of living are low and deprivation is marked. The only exception might be the problems of extreme old age since the poor do not live as long as other groups in society. By living in a well-off community as little as 100 yards away from a deprived area an individual can increase his or her life span by more than 10 years.

Our claim, and that of much research, would be that people and communities living in conditions of poverty and deprivation are much more likely to become vulnerable and need care and protection. This situation is often described as being 'at risk' and it can refer to any client group. Black and ethnic minority groups are often subject to this kind of disadvantage.

It should be emphasised, however, that many people who are not disadvantaged in this way still need the services and support of caring agencies. That is why allocating resources and fixing priorities for the health and welfare services pose such difficult political problems for governments and societies to solve. Which groups deserve the resources that are made available to tackle care needs?

A clear illustration of this dilemma is highlighted by one group of people requiring care – offenders. Offenders present problems to society. Some people think criminals should not be part of the work of caring agencies; they think society's responsibilities should be limited to catching, judging and punishing offenders. This view of criminality suggests offenders should take the consequences for their behaviour and the sentencing of the courts should be seen to deter

others from breaking the law. This view is less useful when we look at the types of people who commit crimes and the impact of sentences on the families of criminals. Many crimes are committed by children and young people; many offenders have histories of mental disorder and chronic illness. Many criminals are responsible for the welfare of others – they are fathers, mothers and carers. The criminal justice system therefore has to be linked to the caring services and offenders themselves often require care as well as control.

When people don't fit in with the expectations of the wider society (sociologists call this 'deviance') then caring agencies are often used to help them and to control their behaviour.

Our list of the people who need care has grown during our discussion – as well as considering vulnerable groups in society we have thought about social conditions and circumstances which make the need for care more likely.

WHO GIVES CARE?

Informal carers

The first group of people who give care are all the informal carers who sustain people needing care in their own homes and communities. Past research has suggested that as much as 90% of all community care is provided by families (spouses/partners, parents, children and other relatives) friends, neighbours and other community supports (such as churches and religious groups). If we do not include ordinary parenting of children as caring work then about 10% of the population will be involved in giving care. About 1-in-4 of these carers will spend over 20 hours a week providing the personal support that people need to continue living in their own homes. A much smaller group can spend almost 24 hours a day looking after other people. The majority of these carers will be women. Caring is a gender issue because it is women who carry out the bulk of the caring work.

Although many carers would not describe their role and responsibilities as a burden it is clear that these kinds of commitments have a huge impact – physically, emotionally, financially and socially – on their lives. Carers are a resource but they also have care needs themselves, and many agencies providing services and benefits are now much more aware of the need to support carers in their role.

Care workers

Although we have acknowledged the immense contribution of informal carers to society, this book is mainly about the other kind of carers – care workers. It is not always easy to work out who they are and how they work to the benefit of clients. This is because of 2 major difficulties – the complexity of care needs and the overlapping roles of many caring organisations and their care workers.

To illustrate these difficulties it is useful to consider an individual with particular care needs, such as Joe.

When you have read the example opposite then try Exercise 3.

● ●

EXERCISE 3

What problems and care needs might Joe and his family have?

● ●

The first problem is the complexity of care needs. Joe's whole world needs to be assessed, with him and his family, to work out the impact of his disability. Each care worker or professional who comes in contact with Joe might only deal with one part of his problems and care needs. Good care workers have to be aware of their own limitations – as individuals and as service providers. They need to know who else to involve and what advice to give service users about other agencies.

Let us look at Joe's world and start to identify some of the issues which have to be tackled. We will try to define a problem or a need and then see who might be able to provide the care or service that could help. We will exclude informal carers like friends and neighbours.

Joe's problems and needs are:

- *Personal care*, **for example, feeding, toileting, lifting, nursing and comforting.**
- *Resources and services* **would include district nurse, health visitor, home help, voluntary organisations, occupational therapist, physiotherapist.**
- *Counselling*, **for example, coping with disability, relationships and sexual problems, depression and loss.**
- *Resources and services* **would include social worker, psychiatrist, community psychiatric nurse, and all the other workers and carers mentioned under personal care.**
- *Physical environment*, **for example, mobility problems coupled with unsuitable housing because of steep hills in area, stairs on the entry and split-level living inside the house.**
- *Resources and services* **would include housing**

> **EXAMPLE**
>
> Joe is in his early 40s and has recently had a stroke. He has been left with serious mobility problems and a speech impairment. He is married with a young family and both he and his wife have had to give up work to concentrate on his care and rehabilitation (a term used by many health and social care professionals meaning to restore a person back to the best level of ability or health that he or she can achieve).

agency and building society, occupational therapist, physiotherapist, social worker, GP and Red Cross.

You probably picked out other needs. These 3 problems and areas of need are not the full picture and within each the resources and services are not an exhaustive list. We could easily pick out other big issues, such as employment and money, to explore.

What emerges quickly on examining Joe's situation is the range of issues and people he and his family have to deal with and the number of agencies and carers with whom they should be linked. One researcher (Blaxter 1980) worked out that a person with a serious disability, living in a town of approximately 100,000 people, could be in contact with as many as 59 agencies. This range is not unusual when people have serious health and social problems in their lives.

Coordination of care is not simple. There is powerful evidence that care workers from different agencies and professional backgrounds define problems and solutions differently.

For example, if Joe's mobility problems are accepted as permanent then the housing agency involved might want him to transfer to a new house. This might disrupt support and the network of informal care the family have nearby. An occupational therapist, however, might want to help Joe learn to walk again and might want to carry out adaptations to the family's home. A more radical view of Joe's world might reject the individual focus on the medical model of making Joe 'better'. Joe's access problems and housing issues would then be defined as society's problem. A disability rights worker would want to involve Joe in fighting for wider reforms and structural change in society, as well as tackling his housing position. (This topic is covered in more detail in *Skills for Caring – Independent Living*.)

2

Key agencies

■ In the government's *Practitioner's Guide on Care Management and Assessment* (HMSO 1991) care needs are described as:

'the requirements of individuals to enable them to achieve, maintain or restore an acceptable level of social independence or quality of life, as defined by the particular care agency or authority.'

This is a helpful approach, but our look at Joe's world emphasised that the views of the person on the receiving end of the caring have to be firmly at the centre of understanding care needs, and that no one agency has a monopoly of resources or understanding of Joe's needs.

Although we have to bear in mind that need is a personal business it can be argued that the main categories of care needs will be the following:

- **personal/social care (including emotional care)**
- **health care**
- **accommodation**
- **finance**
- **education/employment/leisure**
- **transport/access.**

WHICH AGENCIES PROVIDE CARE?

In Chapter 1, we noted that large agencies provided many aspects of health and welfare services, and that social security agencies handled money. We can now begin to develop our understanding of the main sources of provision in the United Kingdom. At this point we will not examine the detailed workings of agencies and organisations, but look at *who* runs the services and *where* the money comes from.

Reading some of this information may seem rather dull, but it is important to remember that, as a care worker, you can be a bank of information for your clients. At times, because of the kind of relationship you have with clients, you might be the only person who is in the right place at the right time to provide key information or advice. By knowing about the fabric of welfare and the roles of agencies you can help prepare clients to use services and get the best results out of the services. Knowledge of the different agencies who provide care also has implications for assessment and care planning.

See Exercise 4.

● ●

EXERCISE 4

Do you know which agencies provide which services and who runs the agencies? When we looked at Joe's situation after his stroke we identified some problems he and his family encountered, including:

- aids and adaptations for his house
- help with Joe's feelings of depression.

Write down which kind of workers could help with these issues and what agencies they would come from. Then identify which part of a government department or authority is responsible for them.

(We will not give you the answer to this exercise because you will discover the possible answers as you read through the chapter.)

● ●

There are 4 key sources of services and resources to help meet the care and welfare needs of people in the United Kingdom:

- Central government and its agencies
- Local authorities and their departments (together the central and local government services are known as the 'public' sector)
- The voluntary sector
- The private sector (sometimes the private and voluntary sector are known as the 'independent' sector).

CENTRAL GOVERNMENT

When we look in detail at the key agencies for social welfare we can consider the impact of the different political systems across England, Wales, Scotland and Northern Ireland on how services are run. In the first instance, however, it is important to identify those services which are the responsibility of central government.

Central government agencies are run by the government of the day – usually the party that won the general election.

See Exercise 5.

● ●

EXERCISE 5

List 3 services that are the responsibility of central government departments.

● ●

The government is made up of ministries and departments which make policies and try to implement them through legislation.

- *Health*
  Central government is directly responsible for the National Health Service. The National Health Service is administered by a range of health authorities in England and Wales, and by boards in Scotland.
- *Social security*
  The government controls and administers the social security system.

The social security system and the Health Service are the main central government agencies we look at in this book. Central government has an indirect responsibility for the personal social services and education which are administered by local authorities. It also has responsibility for the Criminal Justice system (including the Probation Service in England and Wales, and Northern Ireland) and Employment Services.

Employment Services include employment protection and equal opportunities which are safeguards for disadvantaged groups in society. They also run national training agencies and provide counselling and rehabilitation services for longer term unemployed people and for those who have specific health difficulties or disabilities. There are 26 Employment Rehabilitation Centres in operation across the United Kingdom and care workers from different disciplines often work in such centres.

Another role of central government, through development agencies, is the funding and direction of housing associations. Housing associations have become significant partners in social care as they provide services as well as accommodation to client groups with special needs. There are over 2,600 housing associations registered with the Housing Corporation (England), Scottish Homes, and Housing for Wales (similar assistance is available through the Department of the Environment in Northern Ireland).

The housing associations across the country range from small intimate developments to associations with over 10,000 houses on their books. Although their prime goals have been to provide low-cost housing and housing improvement they are part of the strategic development of care in the community. Housing associations are becoming significant employers of care workers and many specialise in support and accommodation for particular client groups, for example, Key Housing for people with learning difficulties, the Richmond Fellowship for mentally ill people, or Margaret Blackwood homes for disabled people. Suitable accommodation with support is often the beginning of discharge from inappropriate hospital care or the vital move to prevent unnecessary hospital admission.

Funding and current issues
One of the features of central government-run services is that a major part of their funding is derived from income tax and national insurance and other sources of government revenue, such as Value Added Tax (VAT). People pay taxes and insurance for most of their working life. This process of contribution explains some of the strong feelings they have about the welfare state and the way it functions. Although agencies funded or run

by government departments may charge for the services they provide, for example, rent for housing association property or charges for dental care, such charges rarely cover the costs of services and are not meant to make a profit or generate income for the government.

The amount of public funds spent on social services, and the relative priority of all public spending against other uses of the country's resources, are issues at the heart of political debate and party differences. We spend as much on defence as we do on education and that is 10% of the country's income. In 1989/90 about 26% of the country's income was spent on social security and 12% on health.

In the early 1980s the government had 2 main objectives in welfare. One was to limit the role of the state, and the other was to control public expenditure (that is, what a government spends). Public expenditure came to over 46% of the country's wealth; by the late 1980s this had fallen to under 40%.

The government philosophy also included the search for the 3 Es – Efficiency, Effectiveness and Economy.

The main thrust of government policy has been to shake up large departments and create smaller agencies with their own budgets and targets for services. There will be over 50 such agencies in the United Kingdom within the next few years. Critics point out that smaller agencies often lead to a reduction in services and inaccessibility, as the offices are centralised and become more remote from the people they serve. There is also concern that the new agencies are not as accountable to parliament as the old departments.

Partly as a response to these issues, the government has introduced a consumer charter movement to ensure standards of services and give people information about their rights.

LOCAL AUTHORITIES

Along with central government agencies and departments the services provided by local authorities are known as the public sector.

A wide range of services is provided by local authorities. Local authorities are councils made up of unpaid elected councillors. There are many types of councils in local government, from Parish Councils and Community Councils to Regional and County Councils. Only the larger kinds of councils provide the public services we are talking about in this book.

In England and Wales (outside Greater London) there are 53 counties and inside them are 369 district councils. The county authorities provide the large-scale local government services like the social services and the police and fire services. In Greater London there are 32 London boroughs and the London City Corporation, along with 5 metropolitan counties which contain 36 district councils.

The rest of the United Kingdom has some similarities to the district and county model but there are differences. Scotland has a 2-tier system and the country is divided into 9 regions with 53 district councils. There are also 3 all-purpose island authorities for Orkney, Shetland and the Western Isles. Northern Ireland has 26 district councils but most services such as housing, education, and health and social services are tied directly to the government, through the Department of the Environment, to the Secretary of State.

> ### SUMMARY OF COUNCIL FUNCTION AND SERVICE RESPONSIBILITY
>
> • County Councils (London Boroughs; Regional Councils in Scotland) Planning; transport; roads/sewage; consumer protection; police/fire; education; personal social services (called social work in Scotland).
> • District Councils
> Environmental health; housing; refuse collection; parks and leisure/recreation; libraries.
> Some services, such as leisure and libraries and parks, vary in the type of council that controls them.

Funding and current issues

In 1988/1989 about a quarter of all central government spending (£42,500 million) was given to local authorities. Although there are some differences between the separate countries in the United Kingdom the funding of local authorities is broadly the same:

- **current expenditure (revenue) comes from government grants, local 'taxes' known as the Rates, Community Charge or Council Tax, and service charges and income**
- **capital expenditure (money spent on buildings and industrial plants) is allocated in a grant from central government or in approval given to borrow monies to complete projects.**

The Block grant (England and Wales) and the Needs grant (Scotland) are meant to subsidise communities up to a recognised level.

The proportion of central government support has been declining over the years. However, over 2,000,000 people are employed by local authorities and nearly half of them are working in education. Present government policy has several significant objectives for the reform of local government, including value for money and accountability.

Value for money
Although local authorities can provide services directly they have been legally obliged since 1988 to contract out or expose certain services to competition. These include refuse collection, catering, vehicle maintenance, ground maintenance and cleaning. It is believed that such competition will provide better value for money and will reduce the expenditure on local government services. The process is known as Compulsory Competitive Tendering. It is likely to be extended to many other areas of local authority services.

Political accountability
Local authority income is derived increasingly from local taxes. The new Community Charge introduced in Scotland in 1989 and England and Wales in 1990 was meant to increase political accountability by making everyone who had a right to vote and use services have responsibility for payment of the tax. Political opposition was fierce and the tax has now been revoked.

Financial accountability
Although the business of local spending and taxation is a local government issue the need to control public expenditure is a central government responsibility. In recent years, the government have introduced a number of measures to inhibit local government spending. All annual accounts are audited by special government appointed bodies and these can take action against local authorities. The government also reserves the right to fix the upper limit that can be set by local authorities for their local tax and also to reduce their grants if they overspend (this is known as 'rate capping').

THE VOLUNTARY SECTOR

Although many people readily recognise certain voluntary organisations, such as Barnardo's, the voluntary sector is rich and diverse and contains all kinds of organisations. A voluntary sector organisation can be defined as a nonstatutory organisation which provides a service or acts in the interests of any client group or groups. Nonstatutory means free from certain legal duties or not set up by law.

It is helpful to think of voluntary organisations in 3 ways:

> - Scale
> - Main purposes
> - Client groups

Scale
When we talk about scale it is usually the level of operation that we're trying to describe. Some voluntary organisations are national and others are local, almost neighbourhood-based. In between, we can have regional and city-based groups. Some voluntary organisations have large numbers working for them and with them, and operate on the world stage, for example, the Red Cross.

Main purposes
The actual purposes of organisations can include a number of activities. The most common are:

- **representing users**
- **representing carers**
- **providing services and care**
- **organising self help**
- **campaigning groups**
- **'umbrella' organisations (coordinating bodies that support organisations, for example, Councils of Social Service or Voluntary, organisations)**
- **representing volunteers.**

Client groups
The list of groups on page 38 covers most of the major client groups but it is important to note that some voluntary organisations are becoming more and more specialised within their areas of interest. For example, care in some organisations of elderly people now focuses particularly on dementia and confusion.

As well as a trend towards special groups or single issue groups there has also been a growth in bodies that specialise in coordinating and linking voluntary organisations, for example, Councils for Social Services, or in running volunteer groups.

Funding and current issues

The role of voluntary organisations in the provision of welfare is increasing. Recent legislation, and the community care movement behind it, have stimulated their growth. The new expansion is partly the result of the enabling duty of local authorities and health authorities, which in turn is partly the result of the government encouraging private sector competition. Local authorities can hold money but do not always have to provide the services themselves. In their enabling role they can buy in services. This means that voluntary organisations are more likely to be involved in partnership agreements with health or social work agencies or have services commissioned by these funding bodies. Many of the recent community care initiatives have involved churches extending their welfare and care roles into a diverse range of projects and services.

Although the large voluntary organisations are not profit-making companies they are in business to make ends meet and sustain services that represent value for money. They can also develop or pioneer new forms of provision or service and operate without some of the pressures of large scale bureaucracies.

Voluntary organisations are funded by many sources. Partnership with health and social welfare agencies provides a contractual model – the funding body, such as a local authority, enters into an agreement to pay for services. This approach should offer some stability to voluntary organisations, as long as they can deliver the commitments at the costs agreed. Traditionally, the voluntary sector has depended on grants from central and local government allied to charges, subscriptions and their own efforts at independent fund raising. Voluntary organisations are very vulnerable to the financial problems caused by what has become known as the 'care gap'. This is the actual difference in cost between providing care and the board and lodgings or income support paid to people who live in care. Without additional monies from local authorities and health authorities many placements would be impossible. This is often described by agencies as planned 'deficit' funding.

See Exercise 6.

• •

EXERCISE 6

What problems do you think voluntary organisations encounter when they try to raise funds from the public?

• •

Fund raising through advertising campaigns can be a problem if the dignity of the client group is damaged and this often causes conflict within organisations. Recently some pressure groups have questioned the portrayal of disabled people as tragic sufferers who deserve pity or charity. The labels used by organisations to describe the focus of their work are also being questioned. For example, 'mentally handicapped' is no longer an acceptable term for many people and alternatives which are less stigmatised are now being used, such as 'people with learning disabilities'.

Voluntary organisations are usually limited by their charitable status in expressing political views or goals, and this can also lead to funding problems if they are considered to be politicised by key funding bodies. Furthermore, there is a limit to the money that ordinary people and bodies can give to charity. Competition for fund raising is fierce. This can stop related organisations working well together for common goals. Central government, health boards or local authorities sometimes find it hard to support organisations which exist, in part, to organise and express criticism of the services they provide.

THE PRIVATE SECTOR

The main type of service provided by the private sector is residential and nursing home care. The same political forces that have expanded the voluntary sector have encouraged the growth of private sector development. The government's belief in market solutions, consumer choice and competition found expression in the Community Care legislation. Both White Papers (a 'White Paper' is a government's proposals for legislation introduced for consultation and discussion) for health and social care emphasised the importance of partnership between private and public sectors. A succession of changes to social security benefit regulations created financial incentives to provide residential and nursing care for a range of client groups. Between 1979 and 1984 the number of residential places provided by the private sector increased by 93%. This has largely been in provision for elderly care clients but there have been increases in provision for mentally ill and handicapped people, and for children and young people. Much of this growth was unplanned and unintended. One of the objectives of community care reform is the control of social security spending on residential and nursing care. One problem that this funding approach created was that residential care became more realistic as a care option than living in the community because there was money to back it. This is one of the central dilemmas that community care reform is meant to tackle.

Within the health service almost 10% of the population is covered by private health insurance. over 500,000 clients a year are treated in private hospitals. The main areas of private health care have been elective surgery, such as hip replacements or coronary artery by-pass grafts, where waiting times for NHS treatment have been lengthy, and hospice care for the terminally ill.

The 'mixed economy' model of social and health care, investing in public, private and voluntary providers of care, will continue to offer opportunities for different types of private service to emerge – the private sector became the major growth employer in health and social care during the 1980s.

Funding and current issues

Private care is funded by a variety of mechanisms including personal disposable incomes and state benefits. Tax relief on insurance schemes and occupational benefits also support the use of the private sector. When individual resources and state benefits do not meet the entire costs of residential or nursing home care, local authorities and health boards and charities often pay a supplement to cover the costs.

The 'Care Element', an important section of the Community Care legislation (in force from April 1993) means that the monies presently held by social security will be transferred to local authorities to purchase residential and nursing home care for people who have made that choice and have been assessed as having those needs. To ensure that local authorities make genuine efforts to use the private and voluntary sector homes the new arrangements for paying social security benefits will not apply to placements in local authority homes. Local authorities will have to meet the full costs of providing residential care if they want to carry on running their own residential services.

3

Where, why, when and how?

■ Chapters 1 and 2 looked at *what* the caring services are and *who* runs them. Chapter 3 considers *where, why, when* and *how* these services are provided.

WHERE DO CLIENTS GET CARE AND SERVICES?

IN THEIR OWN HOMES

It is the view of most agencies, and presumably their consumers, that it is preferable to live in your own home than be cared for in a residential or hospital setting. The most important setting for health and social care to be available to users is therefore in their own homes. Some agencies and parts of services are geared to provide domiciliary support and actively go to the client's home.

See Exercise 7.

● ●

EXERCISE 7

Pick out 3 kinds of service that specifically involve contact with clients in their own homes.

● ●

Your answers to Exercise 7 probably included the following:

• **Within the health service is the primary health care team which often consists of the GP (general practitioner), health visitor, district nurse and, sometimes, other types of care worker such as social workers and occupational therapists. These groups of staff provide services in people's homes.**
• **Social services or social work services are often part of the support given to clients in**

their own homes. Home care provided by care workers like home helps and carers is a central part of maintaining the quality of life and independence of clients.
• **Social contact, respite care (or 'shared care') and practical support are often provided by voluntary organisations, such as Crossroads, the Alzheimer's Society or the WRVS.**

IN OFFICES AND LOCAL BASES

Most health and social care services are run by organisations that have administrative and service bases. These offices are places where referrals can be made but they also provide settings for services, such as information and advice, and group care and support.

IN DAY CARE OR RESOURCE CENTRES

More structured programmes involving day care and therapy for longer periods can be offered in special centres or as part of residential facilities or hospitals.

IN HOSPITALS OR HOMES

Specialist services or services which rely on intense types of care using skilled staff and expensive equipment (such as intensive care and accident and emergency services in the health services) are often located in hospitals, nursing homes or residential units, for example, Spinal Injury Units. Continuing (that is, 24-hour) care is generally offered through homes and hospitals and these vary in scale and style.

The question of where to provide services is tied to values and money. There is a strong belief that many services should be locally available within communities. The principle of accessibility is important within service planning. It is also true, however, that costs have to be taken into account and sometimes it is necessary to centralise services at some distance from communities. This can cause real conflicts, particularly in remote rural areas.

There is also serious debate about whether services should be provided in settings that isolate or segregate groups with special needs. Traditional patterns of service for day care and continuing care have emerged for groups such as elderly people and people with learning difficulties. Creating artificial groups of clients in such settings as training centres or hostels can sometimes reinforce their differences and inhibit their potential to become integrated within the community. On the other hand, it can concentrate expert care and provide services that are uniquely adapted to the client group's needs. The present trend in practice in many agencies embraces **normalisation** as a guiding principle. This approach attempts to ensure that services enhance potential and involve clients in ordinary services and opportunities rather than producing service ghettos that can restrict participation in normal living. You can read more about this approach in *Skills for Caring – Independent Living*.

Now try Exercise 8.

● ●

EXERCISE 8

Some people feel threatened by the thought of people with learning difficulties or a physical disability living next door to them. Why do you think they feel this way?

● ●

The reactions of some individuals and communities to people they think are 'different' can be complicated. When housing associations or local authorities try to plan a project in a local community they often spend time talking to the local community about the project. Some clients resent this kind of consultation. They wonder why building societies don't consult neighbours about the new people before giving mortgages to buy houses.

Local people say different things about the idea of client groups living among them. They often express fears about 'control' and want to know about supervision and fences. They talk about children being frightened by 'difference', and

about the value of their property being affected. There are many similarities to the attitudes that are expressed about black people and ethnic minority groups. Many attitudes are based on the absence of direct experience and knowledge. Unfortunately, the longer society keeps people in isolated long-stay hospitals the longer it will be before communities get the opportunity to understand these citizens.

Access to the range of services available through health and social care agencies is very much a question of how such agencies are organised and how arrangements for assessment of needs are organised. We will look at this question when we consider the main agencies concerned.

One other way of looking at the 'Where?' question involves considering how health and welfare services have a role to play in other kinds of organisations. Within industry and the business world the well-being of employees and the recruitment and retention of staff are important goals for successful performance. Many health and welfare services are located within such organisations to meet the social and health needs of the people who work there. For example, providing crèche facilities for the young children of employees can be helpful to companies.

In the social services themselves the investment by a host agency in other forms of care and support is sometimes a way of tackling and managing problems. The use of social workers in hospitals can free doctors and nurses from time-consuming emotional support work with clients or patients, and coordination of discharge arrangements can help improve the efficient use of beds and the medical team's resources.

Within education settings the use of counsellors and welfare care workers can help reduce problems like truancy and behavioural difficulties because these care workers can make links with families and the community outside the school setting.

In both health and social work settings the employment of occupational health staff can support care workers by helping them to manage stresses created by their work demands. It is now recognised that care workers need care as well as conventional management and supervision. You can find out more about this in *Skills for Caring – Healthy Living*.

WHY PROVIDE SERVICES?

MAKING DECISIONS

The rest of this chapter looks at the debate surrounding the role of welfare in our society.

Before continuing, look at Exercise 9.

● ●

EXERCISE 9

If you held a powerful position as a decision-maker in society how would you make up your mind which needs – from the wide range of priorities and human needs demanding attention and resources – should be given funds? Choose 3 proposals from the following list and give reasons why you think they are important:

• A mass pregnancy screening and genetic counselling programme to identify babies at risk of serious illness or disability.
• A substantial increase in child benefit for all families.
• Every child under 5 years to have access to free preschool nursery care and education.
• Large-scale investment in inner-city areas where there has been unrest because of racial tension and juvenile crime.
• Subsidies for people living in remote rural communities.
• Funding to provide care in the community for AIDS sufferers.
• Benefits for every severely disabled person to employ a full-time personal carer-helper.
• A health education programme targeted at young people, to combat the dangers of smoking, drugs and alcohol abuse.
• Improvements in prison conditions, including better sanitation and a variety of rehabilitation programmes.
• Funding for voluntary organisations to set up supported accommodation in the community for people with learning disabilities and mental illnesses.

● ●

This sort of decision-making is a hard business – whatever is decided has consequences for people in terms of life opportunities and costs. How did *you* arrive at the decisions you made? The judgements we make are affected by the kind of society we have in the United Kingdom, what kind of political

and moral values and beliefs determine our view of human nature, and how we think society ought to be organised.

The United Kingdom is run as a **capitalist system**, with a **market economy** ruled by supply and demand. In other words, individuals and organisations generate income (make money!) and decide how they will spend it. People get rewards for choosing to do things that help society work. The United Kingdom is also a **democracy** – most people have a say in making decisions about society – and it has a **welfare system**. Both these systems try to balance the effects of the competition and inequality which arise from capitalism, by distributing power and resources across society.

Another consideration when making decisions about health and social issues is whether services should be directed at an individual or at society as a whole. This depends on where we think the responsibility for problems and needs lies. For example, Joe's mobility problems (page 6) could be eased by giving him individual aids and adaptations, but if society designed and built a more accessible environment (especially housing and public buildings) Joe could retain his independence with fewer aids.

Different people, including professional groups and agencies, have different views on the causes of human behaviour and health and social problems. Many of the debates about welfare centre round the question of whether people cause their own misery or are unwilling victims of circumstances beyond their control. For example, is crime and delinquency a product of the way society works as well as the result of individual responsibility? Or, if lung cancer is caused by smoking should the treatment of those affected by chronic nicotine abuse be a low priority?

This raises the question of how we judge the extent of a person's responsibility for his or her situation – people may be ignorant of the facts, it may take generations before health problems become apparent; society may be happy to benefit from the income generated by, for example, the tobacco industry; or there may be concerns about restrictions on personal freedom. Societies and political forces make judgements about people and their condition, seeing client groups as 'deserving' or 'undeserving'. The more that blame is attached to individuals for their situation, the more likely it is that the help given has conditions attached to it or is accompanied by expressions of disapproval. The debate about the treatment of people with

AIDS, for example, has raised many of these issues.

You may be thinking, 'What has this to do with the day-to-day tasks that care workers carry out?' More than you realise! These issues are at the heart of the values and attitudes that people as clients and care workers carry into the human exchanges that are the important experiences of welfare. Care workers can either be bewildered by the strength of emotion and aggression displayed by clients in certain circumstances, or disappointed by their depressed and passive attitudes when support is being offered. It can make an enormous difference if care workers are sensitive to the range of underlying feelings that clients can have about being on the receiving end of care.

This is why there is a **Value Base Unit** underpinning the competencies of care. It insists that clients are shown respect and that their emotional needs are met at all times. If clients feel they are a burden on the system, or that their entitlement to service is an admission of personal failure, they will have mixed feelings about care and care workers. One of the challenges of being a care worker is using the opportunities provided by care work to reaffirm a client's sense of worth. How must clients feel if they sit down to cold, unappetising food or are ignored while waiting for a test in hospital? The attitudes of care workers are crucial to care outcomes. (*Skills for Caring – Clients as Individuals* is a helpful source of information on this aspect of care work.)

UNIVERSAL OR SELECTIVE?

Welfare services are generally not given unconditionally. Most social security payments are subject to strict criteria of eligibility or are means tested (that is, assessed on the basis of income). Restricting benefits to certain categories of people is a selective approach. Selective benefits often deter people from claiming assistance and take-up (the number of people entitled to claim) can therefore be low.

Child benefit is an example of a universal benefit – all parents who care for children (and are resident in the United Kingdom) can claim it whether they need it or not. Critics of child benefit suggest it encourages families on low incomes to have children when they can't afford to support them. Supporters say that if it was paid only to the poorest families it would be associated with shame and failure.

See Exercise 10.

● ●

EXERCISE 10

• Point for thought and/or discussion •

What do you think about these 2 approaches – universal and selective – to the provision of services? Are families on low incomes responsible for their situation? Many will be lone parent families, often as a result of widowhood, separation or divorce. Is a woman facing domestic violence 'responsible' if she leaves the marriage or partnership and chooses instead a reduced income, poor housing and limited employment potential because of child care duties? Is her situation anyone's concern but her own?

● ●

Another point to remember when trying Exercise 10 is that benefits and services are more likely to be universal or freely available if they are a short-term measure, for example, maternity benefits are provided for controlled time periods. Long-term benefits attract more conditions and appraisal for continued payment.

One of the ways to balance needs against resources is through the process of redistribution. There are 4 types of redistribution:

- **Over an individual lifetime**
  (for example, retirement is predictable and payment of national insurance gives the right of pension entitlement)
- **Between individuals**
  (for example, people without children contribute towards those families with children)
- **Between present and future generations**
  (for example, investment in training doctors and nurses by one generation secures skills for the next)
- **Between areas**
  (for example, regional aid can be made available to remote communities).

WHEN SHOULD SERVICES BE PROVIDED?

In Exercise 9 one of the problems you had to consider when choosing which proposals received your resources was *when* to intervene in a situation. Is it better, or most cost effective, to provide services that prevent problems or to wait until things go wrong and then step in? The proposals for universal child care provision for preschool children and targeted health promotion campaigns for young people reflect this dilemma.

Try Exercise 11.

● ●

EXERCISE 11

● **Point for thought and/or discussion** ●

Is prevention better than cure? The immediate symptoms or problems that care workers have to deal with can disguise the root cause of the problem. For example, is it more important to tackle the quality of education than the behaviour of truants? Is good health care about the prevention of heart disease or the provision of heart surgery? Should we work with individuals or the communities and systems around them?

● ●

COMPULSORY OR VOLUNTARY?

Decisions also have to be made about whether services and intervention can be left to the choice of individual clients and carers. There are some situations where the law allows independence and choice to be removed from an individual if they are behaving in ways which are likely to cause themselves or others serious harm. For example, those who work in the fields of child care, mental health and with offenders may have to show care for an individual by acting to control him.

There is continual debate about how far the state should be allowed to intervene in people's lives if they or others are at risk. For example, should the police and social services be allowed to remove children from their families if abuse is suspected? It is very difficult to know exactly the degree of risk to children in their own homes, or the state of someone's mental health. However, the use of compulsion usually indicates that the client group have been given high priority, which is why systems and resources have been put in place to protect children and deal with offenders.

HOW IS CARE PROVIDED?

PUBLIC, PRIVATE OR VOLUNTARY?

The proposals put forward in Exercise 9 could be provided through traditional public sector provision, or through the voluntary sector, or through a combination of both. During the 1980s, government increased the role of the private and independent sectors in providing services. This could influence the success of proposals related to particular client groups and social needs because conditions may be applied to the funding and distribution of care and services.

4

The National Health Service (NHS)

■ In 1942 the Beveridge Report set down basic assumptions about the postwar plans for the country's health and social security provision. Beveridge stated that there should be:

'comprehensive health and rehabilitation services for the prevention and cure of disease and restoration of capacity for work, available to all members of the community.'

The report brought to a radical conclusion almost a century of reforms in benefits and health services in the United Kingdom. Acts of Parliament for England and Wales in 1946 and Scotland in 1947 created the now traditional model of the NHS in 1948.

The Acts secured a free service, except for those areas where charges were allowed. The new service required the government to provide accommodation and services throughout the land in the form of hospitals, medical, nursing and other services. It meant the development of specialist care, whether this was to be provided in hospitals, clinics, health centres or in patients' homes. It gave people with money the choice to obtain private care and it allowed doctors to continue private practice for fees alongside their obligation to service the NHS.

It is hard to imagine a society that could deny people access to medical services but this was the situation in the United Kingdom before 1948. Wage earners paid regular contributions to trades unions or other associations and these contributions covered the costs of care in voluntary hospitals as well as family doctors or GPs. Many people could not afford to see a GP when they were ill.

The NHS was an expression of political will that recognised powerful beliefs about society and the interests of different groups. Ill health is inefficient and costly to the community. The more

complex and developed a society becomes the more it needs to deal with disease and illness. Although in our discussion of health in this chapter we want to concentrate on the health services that are directed to individuals rather than public health development, this is not to deny the spectacular achievements over the last two centuries of public and environmental health reforms.

See Exercise 12.

● ●

EXERCISE 12

Talk to someone who has lived through the changes which occurred in 1948 and ask them about health care before the development of the Welfare State. Try to find out what single change made most difference to most people.

● ●

If the NHS was such a wonderful invention why do you think it is now in the throes of yet another wholesale period of reform and transition? The following quote comes from a Secretary of State for Health:

'The NHS is one of the largest civilian organisations in the world. Its staff is growing rapidly. It contains an evergrowing multitude of skills that depend on and interact with each other. It serves an evergrowing range of health needs with ever more complex treatments and techniques. And though the government has made substantial additions to a programme of expenditure which was already planned to grow at an above average rate, there is never enough money – and never likely to be – for everything that ideally requires to be done. Nor, despite the great increases since 1948, are there ever enough skilled men and women.

Figure 2
The reformed NHS

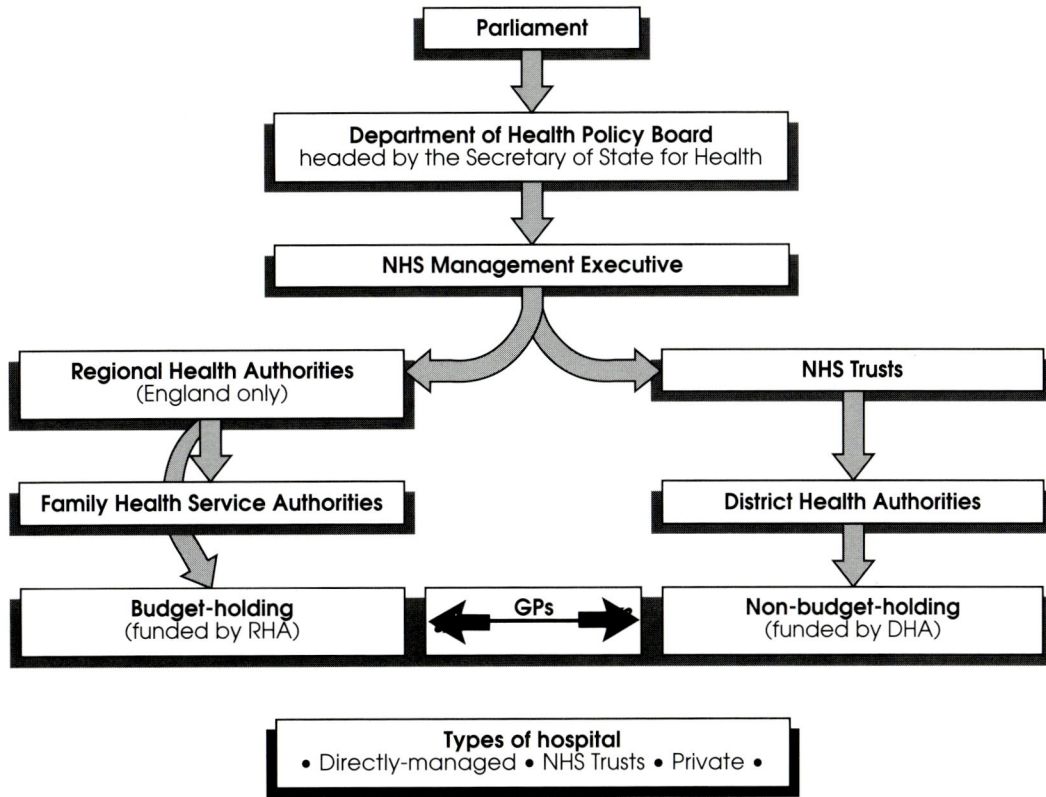

```
                    ┌─────────────────────┐
                    │     Parliament      │
                    └─────────────────────┘
                              ↓
          ┌──────────────────────────────────────────┐
          │   Department of Health Policy Board       │
          │ headed by the Secretary of State for Health│
          └──────────────────────────────────────────┘
                              ↓
          ┌──────────────────────────────────────────┐
          │         NHS Management Executive          │
          └──────────────────────────────────────────┘
                       ↙              ↘
┌───────────────────────────┐    ┌───────────────────────────┐
│ Regional Health Authorities│    │        NHS Trusts         │
│      (England only)        │    │                           │
└───────────────────────────┘    └───────────────────────────┘
              ↓                                ↓
┌───────────────────────────┐    ┌───────────────────────────┐
│Family Health Service       │    │ District Health Authorities│
│Authorities                 │    │                           │
└───────────────────────────┘    └───────────────────────────┘
              ↓                                ↓
┌─────────────────┐  ┌──────┐   ┌───────────────────────────┐
│ Budget-holding  │←─│ GPs  │─→ │   Non-budget-holding      │
│ (funded by RHA) │  └──────┘   │     (funded by DHA)       │
└─────────────────┘             └───────────────────────────┘

          ┌──────────────────────────────────────────┐
          │            Types of hospital              │
          │ • Directly-managed • NHS Trusts • Private •│
          └──────────────────────────────────────────┘
```

Real needs must therefore be identified, and decisions taken and periodically reviewed, as to the order of priorities among them. Plans must be worked out to meet these needs and management and drive must be continually applied to put the plans into action, assess their effectiveness and modify them as needs change or as ways are found to make the plans more effective.

Effective for what? – to improve the service for the benefit of all. The plans must therefore be effective in providing what patients need primarily, treatment and care in hospital; support at home; diagnosis and treatment in surgery health centre or out-patient clinic; or day care. Furthermore, they must include arrangements whereby the public can express their wishes and preferences, and know that notice will be taken of them.

In the final analysis, health care depends on the effective delivery at the right time and place of the skills and devotion of those providing the services required. We are indeed fortunate in this country in the quality of our health teams, and we have good reason to

be proud of the achievement of the National Health Service. Nevertheless, no one would claim that it is perfect.'

This quotation comes from the Foreword to the White Paper on NHS reorganisation, written in 1972 by Sir Keith Joseph. Are you surprised that it was written more than 20 years ago? Are we still trying to solve the same problems?

NHS REFORMS 1991/92

Figure 2 shows how the government's proposals will work. The NHS reforms were laid out in the White Paper *Working for patients* in January 1989. It formed the basis of much of the **NHS and Community Care Act 1990.**

Try Exercise 13 now.

• •

EXERCISE 13

Have a look at Figure 2 and pick out any differences between the old system and the reformed NHS.

• •

There are many changes that could be highlighted:

- **_The creation of a medical market place_**
  The reforms mean that the health service has to split into 2 kinds of entity – purchasers and providers. All hospitals must earn their income by 'winning' or being awarded contracts by District Health Authorities (England and Wales), Health Boards (Scotland), budget holding GPs or from private patients and their insurers. In theory, any hospital can provide the service a patient needs. The system therefore will create competition and this is believed to be a good model for reducing costs and increasing efficiency. If a hospital's services are too expensive they will not attract business and funds will go elsewhere.
- **_Different types of hospital:_**
  There will be 3 kinds of hospital:
  - **directly managed hospitals managed by District Health Authorities or Health Boards, which have to win and keep contracts**
  - **NHS Trusts, hospitals which choose to opt out of direct management**
  - **private hospitals, which are entirely funded by fee-paying patients and users, budget holding GPs or District Health Authorities/ Health Boards.**
- **_Management roles_**
  At the head of the NHS there are powerful new executive posts and teams and all operational services, including Family Practitioner Services, will be under the executive's control.

The government believes that its reforms will help to provide an improved service, while retaining the principle that the NHS is available to all – regardless of income – and financed out of general taxation. Opponents of the system are convinced that it will lead to a 2-tier system which will mean that NHS managers rather than doctors will make choices on business rather than health grounds and that choice for patients will not be a reality. There is also a fear that difficult or 'unattractive' demands for health care will be shifted out of the NHS system into private care, for example, continuing care of elderly people with mental health or behavioural problems. The government insists that such fears are groundless because the NHS will retain ultimate responsibility for the health and care of groups placed in the private sector.

HOW THE NHS WORKS

There are 2 broad categories of health provision – in the community and in hospitals.

Try Exercise 14 before continuing.

• •

EXERCISE 14

Think for a minute about your own health history and that of people you know:

• What different kinds of health care have you been given?
• With which health professionals have you been in contact?

• •

PRIMARY HEALTH CARE

Health care in the community usually means contact with primary health care. Primary health care is provided by doctors, dentists, opticians and pharmacists working as independent practitioners within the NHS, and by health visitors, district nurses, and midwives employed by health authorities or health boards. A wide range of other services are accessible to local communities, such as school health, chiropody, physiotherapy and speech therapy.

For most people health care begins in the community and it is usually the patient himself who decides when and where to seek help or advice. Often, a person's social circumstances and emotional state will have as much to do with a referral as actual physical health problems. This is one of the reasons why health care planning and targeting services can be difficult.

The first point of entry to the NHS will often be an appointment with the patient's own doctor, dentist, optician, or a visit to the pharmacist. Family doctors or general practitioners work in partnerships or group practices (4 out of every 5 doctors) and they often work as members of primary health care teams.

The general practitioner (GP)
The GP is a vital resource within the NHS. Under their contract GPs have to provide health care to the patients on their list. The key elements of this service include immediate and necessary treatment and arranging further treatment from hospitals and other services. GPs are expected to undertake this range of work personally or make deputising arrangements for patients' care.

The system places the GP in a pivotal role for assessment diagnosis and continuity of care. People often turn to their GP to sort out all kinds of personal and social problems as well as health issues. The potentially long-term relationship between GP and patient can become an important channel between people and the services they need.

The character of practices varies with the setting, community and personal style of the GP. In theory, people can exercise choice because they can apply to any GP. In rural areas and some suburban areas, however, the options are limited.

GP training involves 5 or 6 years of undergraduate study, followed by trainee periods of 3 years and supervised practice.

Health visitors, district nurses, midwives

These specialist nurses have special areas of expertise and responsibilities.

Health visitors are responsible for the preventative care and health education of all families, particularly those with young children. They work closely with GPs, district nurses and other professions and agencies such as social workers.

District nurses give skilled nursing care to people at home or elsewhere outside hospitals. They also work on health education and prevention. Most children are now born in hospital but some antenatal and postnatal care is given in the community by midwives.

These specialist community nurses have to train for several years after their 3-year studentship to become a Registered Nurse (RN). In recent years there has been an increase in the number of community psychiatric nurses who work with people who have mental health problems.

The emergence of the nursing profession as significant practitioners and managers within the NHS has been one of the key features of health care. Traditionally, their roles were supportive to doctors. This is still an element of their work but they share considerable responsibility for treatment and supervision of people in the community, particularly those who have long-term health problems. They play an important role in assessment and management of health and social care services provided.

Apart from the early identification of ill health and monitoring of high risk groups, community nurses provide direct care during periods of illness or stress. They often deal with the difficult and painful consequences of illnesses, such as incontinence or pressure sores.

HOSPITAL AND SPECIALIST SERVICES

Most hospital facilities are organised on the basis of a number of considerations. These include specialist focus, geography, training and emergency facilities. During the last century there was a dramatic increase in the number of voluntary hospitals in the United Kingdom. Many of these Victorian institutions still provide care today. Since the beginning of the NHS in the postwar period there has been an attempt to organise the development of hospital facilities to take account of different needs and the costs of providing certain services. Since 1979, over 500 building schemes, across the United Kingdom, most costing £1,000,000 or more, have been completed or started.

See Exercise 15.

● ●

EXERCISE 15

Which hospital services would you expect to find in your local area?

● ●

There are core services which should be available on a local basis. People need local access to the following services:
- **Accident and Emergency (A & E) Departments**
- **immediate admissions to hospital from A&E, for example, general surgery or orthopaedic surgery**
- **other immediate admissions, for example, psychiatric services or general medicine**
- **out-patient support for all these types of care.**

Then there are specialist services which might not be available in every area but which might be based on a regional, supraregional or national basis, for example, heart and liver transplants, renal (kidney) units and intensive care for newborn children.

Most hospitals will fall under one or more of the following categories:

- **teaching hospitals**
- **regional hospitals**
- **general hospitals**
- **hospitals for specific diseases, for example, eye, skin or infectious disease**
- **long stay/continuing care, for example, care of elderly people or young chronically sick people**
- **mental hospitals.**

21

Medical staff are organised within hierarchical clinical teams in hospitals. In former times, the medical staff used to be known as 'firms' under the control of a specialist or consultant. Although consultants and their teams (senior and junior registrars, senior and junior house officers) still have clinical responsibility for patients in the various units or specialist setting, nursing staff, who are managed separately, have become increasingly involved in procedures previously carried out by doctors, for example, obstetrics and intensive care. The power base within hospitals has also shifted away from clinicians towards managers who are accountable for overall performance to the Regional Authority or the Health Executive.

See Exercise 16.

● ●

EXERCISE 16

Try and list the different kinds of specialists or consultants who might be found in NHS hospitals.

● ●

How many specialisms did you manage? There are probably well over 30 different kinds of specialism but, generally, they are grouped according to particular parts or systems in the body, techniques of interventions (such as surgery or rehabilitation), age stages in life, or stages in the identification and treatment of illness. Some of the more common areas of specialism are shown in the panel on the right.

We have already touched on some of the problems associated with this way of organising medical services. There is the problem of reductionism – if we define people and their problems as specific parts or systems of their bodies we might lose out on understanding the whole person and their health problems. People often have more than one kind of health problem and some disorders present multiple health problems. That is why assessment and cooperation between health professionals and other professions and care workers are important.

Other workers in the hospital services

A range of occupational or professional groups in central departments, or attached to specialist units, provide additional support and services for patients. The level of independence they exercise in relation to cases depends on the health problems involved or their role in the clinical team. Doctors

---

COMMON AREAS OF SPECIALISM

- Audiology – the study of hearing and assessment of deafness
- Geriatrics – specialised study of disorders of middle age and beyond, and their treatment and management
- Neurology – study of diseases of the nervous system, including epilepsy and brain injuries
- Paediatrics – study of child health and diseases (neonatology is concerned with newborn children)
- Psychiatry – study of mental disorders which can include mental illnesses and serious learning difficulties, however they are caused
- Genetics – study of heredity and how diseases are inherited
- Orthopaedics – surgery connected with correcting injuries and deformities of the skeleton (bones)
- Urology – study and treatment of diseases of the urinary tract
- Cardiology – study of heart and circulatory diseases
- Dermatology – study and treatment of disorders of the skin.

---

are often thought by these other groups to be ill-informed about their contribution to the welfare of patients and their carers. This can result in inappropriate referrals and confusion about roles.

Sometimes, the groups are known as auxiliary groups. Their development has often been a struggle for professional status and recognition within the medical world. The main groups are shown in the panel on page 23.

The functions, organisation, training and pay of all these groups have often been the subject of national studies and committees. They all have systems of training and bodies which award qualifications. Apart from social workers all the groups are recognised as supplementary medical professions and they can obtain registration for their training which lasts from 1-4 years depending on the group. Only registered practitioners can be employed in the NHS and other public services.

In addition to these occupational groups there are other helpers, such as ambulance personnel (the Ambulance Service is run by independent national organisations) and the Blood Transfusion Service.

The NHS is the largest employer in the United

PROFESSIONAL GROUPS

- Chiropodists – treat problems in feet and hands
- Dieticians – give special advice to doctors and patients about diet, and support patients to pursue healthier eating habits; also help with research for diagnosis and treatment and have a broad interest in promoting health education and training
- Technicians – use instruments, tests, and data to help clinicians diagnose, treat, or study illness
- Occupational Therapists – work towards the psychological, physical, and social rehabilitation of patients: this can involve activities, technical help with aids and adaptations, and counselling; both mental and physical health problems are tackled
- Physiotherapists – treat by physical means, such as heat, light, electricity, massage, and movement; treatment can be part of the preparation or recovery from other interventions, such as before and after major operations, but it also covers a wide range of illnesses, including problems with bones and joints, and neurological illness

- Orthopticists – investigate, diagnose and treat squints and other defects using exercises and instruments; their measurements are also used to plan and assess the results of delicate surgery to the eye
- Radiographers – use X-ray pictures to help diagnose conditions
- Speech Therapists – concerned with the assessment and treatment of speech disorders that might include articulation (getting the words out), language use, such as not understanding written forms of communication, voice problems, perhaps after removal of the larynx, and fluency, such as stammering; often work with other carers to help them develop their own training skills and understanding
- Psychologists – clinical psychologists and educational psychologists try to measure, assess and evaluate psychological behaviour and functioning; they are also involved in treating conditions using a range of methods, such as behaviour therapy or counselling
- Social Workers – offer counselling and problem-solving skills as well as providing a range of practical supports and advice about other welfare systems and services.

Kingdom. About 50% of its employees are nurses and over 7% are doctors. The rest include a large number of care workers and domestic staff. Different levels of training are required for these support roles.

Whether patients are seen on an inpatient or outpatient basis the facilities and services provided by the whole range of helping professionals attached to hospitals should be available when needed.

The voluntary sector

Within NHS hospitals many well-known voluntary organisations, such as the Red Cross and Women's Royal Volunteer Service, run services to provide essential comforts and supports to patients and their carers. In addition, almost every major illness or disease has self-help groups and organisations devoted to the welfare of sufferers and their informal carers, for example, the Multiple Sclerosis Society or the Epilepsy Association. In recent years, these groups have become more influential as sources of consultation with representative groups of patients and service users.

DOES THE NHS WORK?

We posed this question when we looked at the structure and funding of the health service: the major political parties have different analyses of the problems and different solutions. There is, however, reasonable agreement about the need to have good access to effective medical care.

QUALITY ASSURANCE AND FUNDING

This has emerged as an important theme in the NHS. For some political parties the main contribution to quality would be an increase in funding support from central government linked to the establishment of locally available services. Government critics point out that the level of spending on health in the United Kingdom has not kept pace either with other European countries or with the United States of America.

The government has countered this criticism with the view that real gains will be produced by more effective management and by increasing competition and consumer control. To achieve this they have introduced various measures to improve the health service, including:

- **the encouragement of private sector provision and private insurance to reduce demand on the public sector purse**
- **the creation of a Citizen's Charter (or Patient's Charter) for health services that spells out standards and gives the kind of information people need to know if they wish to complain, for example, waiting times, standards of premises and choice of hospitals**
- **the move towards a purchaser/provider split that allows NHS managers and GP fund holders to get value for money by contracting services to the best source for value and quality, and keeps these issues in front of managers when they evaluate the return they get for the money spent**
- **the allocation of specific grants from the government to health authorities and health boards (often in partnership with local authorities) to develop special facilities and services; the government can check on the progress of such schemes and reward achievement.**

Critics, however, argue that the reforms have deflected the NHS from its main goal and will waste resources. The Citizen's Charter is seen as ineffective because it gives no new rights to people and the actual democratic accountability that used to be part of the NHS through representative health boards or authorities has been undermined. The present system for complaints (the Health Service Ombudsman) is only applicable to hospital services and does not cover GPs.

Only through systematic research and the passing of time will we know whether the patients and their carers have benefited from the changes.

FUTURE CONCERNS

POVERTY

Despite the consensus around reports such as the Black Report (HMSO 1980) there is still inadequate recognition of the role of poverty and inequality in health and health provision. Health care still does not reach those most in need.

COORDINATION AND COLLABORATION

Many serious government reports, like the Court Report on Child Care (DHSS 1976), the Jay Report on Mental Handicap Nursing and Care (HMSO 1979), and the Warnock Report on Special Education Needs (HMSO 1978), have highlighted the fragmentation of services and professionalism in health and welfare. Critiques of services within the present community care reforms identify the same concerns about a wasteful absence of joint planning and service delivery.

There has to be a serious examination of the jobs that need to be done for many groups of disabled and chronically sick people. Jay and Warnock pointed to the need for common training rather than separate professions. It is time that agencies and professions worked out how to work together.

At a local level, GPs are the gatekeepers to many benefits and services. In the new community care arrangements local authority social services and social work departments will be the lead agencies for care assessment and management of individual care packages. Apart from money and resources, attitudes and levels of cooperation will have to be improved to make this system work.

ETHICAL CONCERNS

Life and death issues have taken on a new meaning for health professionals and care workers. Medical advances have created new dilemmas for health care. Life can be started artificially and can be prolonged artificially, and through genetic engineering life's future potential can be predicted and controlled. Each new technical procedure or discovery poses questions for society to answer. Care workers in many situations will have to face the consequences of such decisions and policies as carers and as citizens.

ENVIRONMENTAL ISSUES

Health is still viewed as a personal business but the structures and systems of modern industrial society create ill health. We have already looked at the link between substance abuse (cigarettes and alcohol) and economic pressures (jobs and taxes). There are other big scale problems such as traffic, transport and pollution which present health consequences. Preventative health education is aimed at changing individual lifestyles not at changing the world. In any case, it represents a small portion of the resources devoted to health care. Health education priorities for the 1990s are heart disease, smoking, alcohol and drug misuse, cancer, AIDS, dental health and accidents. The tone is one of encouragement rather than prescription.

5

Social security

CASH BENEFITS AND WELFARE

Social security is unlike any other kind of service we have talked about in this book. The service is not a personal one delivered by people like doctors or care workers. It often comes in the form of cash benefits and the social security system in the United Kingdom is entirely the responsibility of central government. The Department of Social Security is run by civil servants on a nationwide basis. Even Scotland has the same system as other parts of the United Kingdom in that the Scottish Office has no minister responsible for social security. Like every other part of the Welfare State the present system has recently undergone significant change and reform.

See Exercise 17.

● ●

EXERCISE 17

A basic understanding of the benefit system is essential for all carers and care workers. Why do you think this is?

● ●

Almost every decision made about the care and welfare of clients has financial implications. Options for care and placements are often decided on the basis of availability of cash benefits or the consequences for individual entitlement to benefits. It is part of the care worker's role to understand the benefit system, or at least know where to get advice and information about benefits. A care worker with a good working knowledge of cash benefits can help a person or a family increase their income by encouraging and supporting them to claim benefits at the right time. Some simple reference

books about cash benefits are recommended at the end of the book.

The stated aim of the social security system is to provide an adequate and responsive system of financial support for all those people who need and are eligible for financial help. In developed societies, money is the key resource people use to meet basic human needs like food, shelter and clothing. It is also the resource that people need to take an active part in society and to meet their obligations as carers and providers for themselves and others. Almost all care and welfare is a balance between provision by families and by the state.

In Chapter 1 we identified a range of vulnerable groups in society who are not able to provide for themselves without help. These groups include people who are elderly, sick, disabled, unemployed, widowed, or bringing up children. Most people in these groups find that their opportunity to work and earn income is limited or curtailed. We noted that some experiences and conditions of incapacity are time limited, for example, maternity, but others, such as learning difficulty, can be lifelong. We also considered who was responsible for dependency and a person's problems. In some situations, people could be judged to have created their own problems, for example, criminals, and this affected how society considered what kinds of support and help should be made available to them. Within our culture there is a strong feeling, called 'the work ethic', that people should work for a living and pay their way. One by-product of this belief is that some benefits are paid at higher rates to people who have worked and, therefore, contributed by paying their National Insurance.

This gives us some indication of some of the difficulties society faces in trying to work out a fair and reasonable system of social security benefits.

25

KEY FEATURES OF THE SOCIAL SECURITY SYSTEM

The national cost of cash benefits is high. The present British system accounts for over 30% of all government expenditure and it has doubled in cost since 1970. The costs continue to rise. The basic structure of the social security system was established nearly 50 years ago. There are 2 main kinds of benefit: contributory and noncontributory. Contributory benefits are paid from the National Insurance fund which consists of contributions from employed people and their employers, self-employed people, and the government. This group of benefits includes retirement pensions and sickness benefits. Noncontributory benefits, such as income support, are financed from general taxation.

A number of noncontributory benefits have special conditions attached to them. Some are means tested, that is, they are income related. To get the benefit a person has to prove that he or she qualifies by not having too much money already as income or sometimes as capital, for example, savings. Other noncontributory benefits depend on meeting particular conditions, for example, having children, or having mobility problems through disablement.

The social security system is set up to ensure that all citizens have adequate means to support themselves and their dependents. Many critics and claimants consider that the system has failed to achieve this central objective. They have this view because poverty is still a widespread concern and many benefits do not appear to reach the groups of people who are entitled to them.

DOES SOCIAL SECURITY WORK?

To find out whether the system is effective or not we need to establish a measure of performance – some benchmarks for judging success. The present system owes much to the Beveridge formula. The Beveridge Report (HMSO 1942) was a bold statement that shaped much of the Welfare State in post war Britain. One of Beveridge's goals was the eradication of poverty – 'freedom from want'. But how was the poverty level to be worked out?

Try Exercise 18 now.

EXERCISE 18

Make some brief notes on what you mean by 'poverty'. When you can, ask 2 friends what they think poverty is and compare their ideas with yours.

Beveridge's key idea was the guarantee of a subsistence income, the minimum required to live. This approach was influenced by research carried out by the great reformer B.S. Rowntree. He studied poverty in surveys stretching into the 20th century and produced statistics on poor people and their income levels, developing the idea of a 'poverty line'. He also offered information on the costs of physical survival.

Beveridge concluded that there are 2 main causes of poverty: interruption or loss of earnings, for example, through unemployment or old age, and low wages, that is, wages that don't meet families' needs. He proposed a redistribution of money from those who worked to those who could not (social insurance) and he wanted money from individuals and small families to go to larger families (childrens' allowances).

The third element of Beveridge's proposals was the creation of National Assistance. This was designed to provide a subsistence income for people not covered by National Insurance or private insurance. In these cases people might not have paid their full level of contributions over time or their entitlement to benefit might have run out. Also the level of benefit set might not meet the special needs of large families or people with serious health problems.

The problems that faced Beveridge's scheme are still with us. He had to persuade the Treasury to set a reasonable level of benefit. He had to produce a benefit system that took account of a changing world. For example, he grossly underestimated how many lone parents there would be in Britain. He never managed to influence the Treasury to set realistic levels of benefits. This meant that the limited scheme of National Assistance became the most important element of income maintenance. Almost all the families receiving National Insurance also had to claim National Assistance. Part of the problem related to the government's reluctance to raise benefit levels to a point where people might be unwilling to work for a living. This is often described as 'maintaining the incentive to work'. This is the modern version of the 'less eligibility' test applied by the 19th century Poor Law. People in need faced the prospect of the workhouse if they claimed assistance, which often meant the break up of families and life in an institution.

The government of the time, 1945, trimmed Beveridge's proposals. Family Allowance was only paid for the second child and the actual benefit levels fell far short of the Beveridge recommendations. The legislation which implemented the Beveridge proposals was part of the reform package that developed the idea of the Welfare State. The legislation on social security failed to tackle longstanding tensions built into the system of social security.

Over the years, the benefit system has failed to meet its central objective because the money available for benefits has never been enough to tackle individual and family poverty. Definitions and debates about poverty levels have been a constant feature of social administration and politics in this country. The definition mentioned earlier (page 5) was offered to researchers in a welfare rights project (Casserly & Clark 1978) by a disabled woman and sums up the client's view: 'I've too much of the week left at the end of my money'. This crushing reality is faced by many of the most vulnerable groups in our society. Structural problems in the economy, such as loss of traditional industries, have created mass unemployment at different stages in the country's economic development. When people are deprived of work they claim benefits; long-term dependence on benefit creates poverty.

See Exercise 19.

● ●

EXERCISE 19

How many poor people do you think live in the the United Kingdom today?

● ●

Poverty was rediscovered in the 1960s by researchers like Townsend and Abel Smith. At first, they followed the old model of pricing the cost of living, comparing this to benefit rates and income levels, then working out how many people in what types of groups were 'poor'. They estimated that 7,500,000 people in the United Kingdom lived in poverty. This finding came at a time when the country was experiencing the 'never-had-it-so-good' era.

Later research tried to redefine poverty as more than subsistence levels: it was also not being able to participate in normal living in society. Poverty was identified as one aspect of the deprivation characterised by poor housing conditions, low levels of health and restricted life style often imposed on entire communities. For example, should benefit levels be set high enough for people to be able to afford newspapers or television rental, or visit other people, or drink or smoke? Townsend (1979) concluded that poverty was not an absolute concept or idea – all human needs including food were, he argued, conditioned by the society in which people live.

In 1966, the government introduced the **Supplementary Benefit Act** to help remove some of the bad feelings associated with the National Assistance Board (NAB). But the old problems remained, despite the different title. People often feel ashamed to claim benefits, particularly means-tested benefits. Not claiming benefits is a serious cause of poverty. The benefit called 'Income Support' is the level of income most often used to describe where the poverty line is.

Clearly, the question about how many people live in poverty (Exercise 19) is difficult to answer simply. Not only is it difficult to define poverty but also governments do not like to admit that there are large numbers of people living in poverty. This means that information is not kept nationally that directly comments on poverty as defined by Income Support levels. Social Trends (Central Statistical Office 1991) tells us that over 4,500,000 people claimed the safety net benefits of Income Support and Family Credit. These people are often part of a household with dependents. The number of people living in poverty is likely to be much higher.

Strathclyde Regional Council is one of a number of local authorities which do keep track of poverty. The Council found that 20% of the region's population lived at or below the poverty line and that 1-in-4 children and elderly people lived in poverty. These figures are not remarkable for large urban areas and rural communities. People in poverty are not just numbers. It should be remembered that the most vulnerable groups in society actually need more money than others. The 20% of people with the lowest household income include:

- **pensioners – 25%**
- **disabled – 5%**
- **unemployed – 27%**
- **low paid – 26%**
- **lone parents – 8%**

(From: Social Trends 1992)

This isn't much different from the situation Beveridge set out to change in 1942. There is a major difference in the distribution of wealth across the population. The percentage of wealth owned by the groups at the top end is growing. The most wealthy 25% own 75% of the country's wealth. This makes the relative poverty of poorer groups more obvious.

Try Exercise 20 whenever you have time.

● ●

EXERCISE 20

Find out how people of different ages feel about claiming benefits. Talk to someone from each of these age groups – 20s, 30s, 40s, 60s and 80s. Ask your older clients about life before benefits and the NHS.

● ●

Children must be fed well. Elderly and severely disabled people need extra warmth and adequate diets. Lone parents need to pay for child care. People with serious mobility problems have to pay for personal transport. Almost every aspect of vulnerability translates into economic cost as well as personal cost. It is difficult to believe that our income maintenance system does work if a fifth of the people are very poor and they include the most vulnerable groups in our society.

See Exercise 21.

● ●

EXERCISE 21

What are the biggest barriers that stop people getting the cash benefits to which they are entitled? (This problem is often described as low 'take-up'.)

● ●

There are 3 main problems which cause low take-up:

- Stigma
- Ignorance
- Complexity

STIGMA

Despite the continual efforts of social security and welfare agencies to improve their image people often feel a deep sense of shame about claiming benefits. Although social insurance is well understood people still have mixed feelings about claiming benefits. Here are the experiences of some claimants:

'I always leave my legs off when the Social Security officer visits, I feel like a sponger but at least they see what's wrong with me' (disabled man who lost both legs in an accident).
'I pulled the chair to get nearer the counter but it was bolted to the ground. I didn't want anyone to hear my business but when the chair wouldn't move I felt ashamed' (lone parent in an old DHSS office).

These people were not exercising rights as citizens in a confident manner – they did not *feel* like customers. Poverty, however it is caused, erodes self-confidence and self-esteem. When people claim benefits they expose themselves to scrutiny and assessment. The acceptance of their claim depends on their low status as workers, providers or whole persons.

Stigma means having a 'spoiled identity' (Goffman 1968) and being stereotyped by other people as undesirable. This could include being discriminated against. People with visible attributes, such as race, colour or disability, often experience prejudice and discrimination.

You can read more about this in 2 other *Skills for Caring* books, *Independent Living* and *Clients as Individuals*. People with other forms of disadvantage can feel that others consider they have a 'spoiled identity', for example, unemployed people, lone parents or criminals. They can experience assessment for benefits as a potential threat to their status. Within the benefits system there are many hurdles which test claimants and make them feel unsure about their self-worth. Many benefits depend on medical assessments; others depend on assessment of income. These processes of assessment can be intrusive and demanding. If a claim is refused people often feel that they have been mistrusted and not believed. The risks to self-esteem and the low value of some benefits can mean that people don't pursue claims or appeals.

IGNORANCE

Many claimants do not apply for benefits because they are unaware that they have an entitlement. People often become involved in the benefit system because of changes in their lives. Such changes can sometimes be traumatic, particularly bereavement, retirement, redundancy, discharge from long-term institutional care and illness. At these times, people often are not at their best at making decisions, following up information or asserting themselves. If they also lack a basic knowledge of rights and systems it is easy to see why claims are not made.

Many benefits have limits on back-dating, that is, getting paid for any period of entitlement before a claim has been made. Up until the late 1970s it was even difficult for claimants to know how the benefits and pensions they received were made up, which is like a working person not having a payslip. This is also important because of the high number of mistakes made by Department of Social Security (DSS) in individual cases. The Audit Commission has criticised the DSS for high percentages of inaccuracy in claims.

In recent years, the methods used to publicise information about benefits have changed and have also included the systematic use of television advertising. However, there is still a tendency to use high profile campaigns for those benefits which attract public sympathy, such as disability rights, or which support the work ethic, such as family credit for working parents. Many other benefits are not advertised in the same way. One helpful way of presenting information is the grouping of all financial information under a client group headline, for example, 'Benefits for Lone Parents', and this approach has become more common.

See Exercise 22.

● ●

EXERCISE 22

Next time you visit a Post Office try and find as many up-to-date leaflets as you can about benefits.

● ●

One positive way to help clients get the benefits they should be receiving is to offer support to them in claiming, either by finding out about the benefits or helping clients to complete forms. Most people need support and representation if they try to appeal against decisions made by social security offices.

COMPLEXITY

Apart from the fact that there are so many benefits – well over 30 major ones – they tend to interact with each other to cause complications. They can cause what is called a 'poverty trap', when

claiming one benefit reduces the value of another or has an effect on wages and taxes. There is also obvious inequality at times when the levels of benefit and conditions of award vary unfairly, even though the needs involved may be the same. A disabled person born with a life-long disability is treated differently from someone injured in an accident at work. This is difficult for people to understand or accept.

Major benefits are also provided and administered through different systems. The Inland Revenue (income tax assessment) and the local authorities (Housing Benefit, Community Charge/Council Tax rebate and educational benefits, such as free school meals) also provide, directly or indirectly, benefits to people. All of this has to be meshed into the overall system of the DSS. So it is not surprising that people don't always understand how it all works.

Social security benefits themselves have varied conditions for eligibility and decision making about entitlement. Benefits can be:

- **taxable or not taxable**
- **treated as income for other benefits or disregarded**
- **contributory and nonmeans tested**
- **noncontributory and nonmeans tested**
- **noncontributory and means tested**
- **discretionary**
- **based on medical assessment**
- **open to appeal**
- **open to review.**

Individual claimants and their families can be involved with all of these systems. It is not surprising that people find them complicated and often fail to get the benefits they need and which they are due.

PAST AND PRESENT

There has been concern in recent years about the level of public expenditure being committed to providing benefits and the impossibility of controlling their growth.

See Exercise 23.

● ●

EXERCISE 23

We established earlier that monies spent on benefits by the country were rising. Why do you think this is the trend?

● ●

There are many reasons why the amount spent on benefits is increasing but 2 of them deserve comment. Firstly, the number of people in certain high risk groups is increasing, for example, there are more elderly people living alone, more lone parents with dependent children, more divorced people, more births outside marriage and more unemployed people.

Secondly, certain features of the social security system set up after 1966 had built-in cost factors:

- **Benefit uprating, which is usually but not always done every year, was based on wage increases. This was generally higher than prices.**
- **Many of the basic benefits, such as Supplementary Benefit, could have additions and other discretionary payments added to them depending upon needs, for example, extra heating for housebound people. All of these decisions were subject to rights of appeal before independent tribunals. It was easier to establish grounds for additional payments in such a scheme.**
- **The staffing costs required to process the complex and overlapping systems of benefit were high.**

The government's response to many of these problems was worked out during the 1980s in 'The Fowler Review' (named after the Secretary of State, Sir Norman Fowler). The **Social Security Act 1986**, which followed the review, was implemented in 1988. The main changes introduced were the replacement of Supplementary Benefit with Income Support and the Social Fund and the development of the Family Credit benefit to take over from Family Income Support. Housing Benefit was also changed.

It is important to understand the implications of changes from the different points of view of those involved in the system. What the Government saw as an achievement the critics and claimants regarded as cuts. The reforms certainly attempted to streamline administration in that the same system and conditions for calculating benefit apply to most of the major means tested benefits – Income Support, Family Credit and Housing Benefit but they are still based in separate administrative systems.

The government's objective in controlling expenditure has often been described by ministers as the need to target benefits to those most in need. The other view is that they want to cut the number of people receiving such assistance. Within the

1986 Act a number of groups were excluded from the system. Students were no longer able to claim benefits and young people between 16 and 18 were also taken out of the benefit system (unless they satisfy special criteria).

For many claimants and their families, the old system had provided a meagre lifeline through the discretionary additions that could be claimed, for example, on Income Support (exceptional additions or single payments). All this was changed. From the government's side the system was unfair and led to inconsistency. The rules for such payments became much stricter and subject to time limits and budgets for local offices – the client might have the need but the office didn't have the money. The scope provided at tribunals to argue for rights was curtailed and appeals could only be based on points of law. Another feature of the Social Fund, which now gives out the grants, was that the payments could be made on the basis of interest free loans (Crisis Loans). This naturally depresses demand for the benefit but does not diminish the needs that claimants experience. If you do not have enough money to buy new shoes for your children it is a 'crisis' but the style of the benefit is unlikely to encourage you to claim for it as one. There may be a worse crisis next week and you would not be eligible for help if you had already committed yourself to a loan.

The Community Care Grant is also administered by the Social Fund. This grant is given to priority groups of claimants who might be moving out of care, hospital or prison to set up a new home. There are also grants for families under pressure. The labelling attached to these benefits is unhelpful and degrading. The normal level of grant is £500. This is hardly a generous level but the recognition that financial support is needed to integrate within the community is helpful and the Commissioner for the Social Fund can be used to review decisions made by local Social Fund Officers.

During these processes of change the rights of claimants have been protected, supposedly, by schemes of transitional protection.

The next phase of the evolution of the social security system is currently underway. In 1988 the government published the 'Next Steps' initiative. This sets out to create separate agencies for different parts of the social security benefit system. The changes move benefits into a model of customer services and disengage the social security departments from direct parliamentary control. In April 1991 the Department of Social Security became the Social Security Benefits Agency

(SSBA) and the other agencies planned or introduced are the Resettlement Units Agency (dealing with homeless and rootless people), the Information Technology Services Agency (already significant levels of work are contracted out to private contractors) and the Child Support Unit (this agency starts off where the old 'liable relatives' section used to operate in trying to force relatives, usually fathers in desertion, to pay maintenance for children).

These agencies represent a major image shift for social security in that their organisation reflects a business model and targets for achievement focus on customer care and efficiency in processing claims. They will work to defined cash limits rather than discovering and meeting needs. This approach complements the strategy the government launched with the Citizen's Charter, aimed at 'raising the standard'. What impact it will have remains to be seen.

THE ROLE OF CARE WORKERS

Throughout this overview of the social security system we have tried to emphasise the link between money and care. There are benefit issues for all the main client groups. There is a constant role for care workers in understanding the need of client groups and the changing system of benefits. For example, in 1993 there will be key changes in benefits for all seriously disabled people. With the introduction in April 1993 of the DSS aspects of the Community Care legislation the monies paid to clients will become part of the costs of care. It will be necessary to understand those elements of statutory benefits, like Income Support and the Social Fund, which will be used to meet the care needs of clients.

Another significant change has occurred in the benefits for disabled people. The **Disability Living Allowance** and **Disability Working Allowance Act** went through Parliament in June 1991. They came about after many years pressure from disability rights groups and other organisations and the government's own survey of the needs of disabled people (OPCS Survey 1988/89). The old Attendance Allowance and Mobility Allowance are being replaced by the new benefits and the role of medical assessment is being reduced. These benefits at 1991 levels were worth more than £70 per week to a disabled person. Although the reforms have been criticised as not tackling the real financial needs of clients these benefits can still make a difference to the quality of life for many people.

Care workers can help with benefit issues on 2 levels. Firstly, they can make sure they know enough to put clients in touch with information and advice and, secondly, they can support clients in actually claiming benefits. Apart from the direct benefit such knowledge can bring to clients, the care demonstrated in knowing and doing something about rights can help create good working relationships with clients.

6

The personal social services

■ There is a general vagueness about the idea of the personal social services, or social work as it is called in Scotland. In this chapter we describe the tasks and roles of social work and social services and indicate some of the main features of the settings and organisational context of social work. Goldberg and Warburton (1979) talk about the 'vastness and vagueness' of social work. They suggest that 50 years after the introduction of systematic training for social workers, colleagues in other disciplines, such as doctors and nurses, often 'ask in exasperation ... what do they do?' This chapter tries to provide answers to that question and also to highlight the work and contribution of a range of care workers associated with social service and social work departments.

BACKGROUND

In earlier chapters we noted that most social services are provided through local government-run departments. These are large scale organisations. They are often called the statutory services because they have to carry out a range of tasks and functions, like child protection, that are laid down in law by Parliament.

Modern day social services owe their shape and organisational style to reorganisation that was carried out at the beginning of the 1970s. In both England and Wales, and in Scotland, there were government appointed inquiries into welfare services that led to recommendations that the various independent social care and welfare agencies should be amalgamated to form new departments run by local authorities. The reasons behind these significant policy shifts were:

- *Client needs*
  Troubles seldom come singly. Many social problems are complex mixtures of personal and social difficulties. Although clients might be labelled as 'offenders' or 'truants' or 'mentally ill' they often had similar problems. It was unhelpful to have a succession of workers from different agencies visiting and working with the same families and clients.

- *Efficiency*
  There was a shortage of trained staff and it was pointless to have the probation service, the mental health service, the children's departments, and the school welfare services (plus all the voluntary agencies) chasing the same limited group of qualified staff. If the services combined then the resources that could be brought to bear on families' and communities' problems would be much greater.

- *Service development*
  It was recognised that clients, groups, families and communities needed to be understood in a wider context than individual circumstances. They also needed services that were locally based, coordinated and accessible to clients and other agencies. Services were to be organised around community needs on an area-based model. This was often called the 'single door' approach.

It was hoped that the new services would be able to tackle unmet needs and develop new approaches to long-standing social problems.

All the different kinds of social workers and carers were using the same basic skills. By uniting the professional groups and the agencies it was also possible to bring together the training resources to create a new jointly recognised professional qualification, the **Certificate of Qualification in Social Work (CQSW)**. It was later joined by the **Certificate in Social Services (CSS)** and these are the main sources of professional status in social work. These qualifications were described as generic training as opposed to the older specialised forms of courses that were used to train groups such as children's officers or mental health officers.

The new departments were accountable to local committees of elected members and were run by directors of social services on social work. They were organised largely on the basis of territorial or political boundaries. The area-based services were provided through area teams and these often had a community focus. Sometimes these area teams and sub-teams might be known as patches.

During the last 20 years the scale of these departments has increased dramatically. As well as area teams, services for residential and day care users have been developed. In some authorities, services in these residential settings were run centrally from administrative headquarters. In most authorities, additional specialist teams have been formed to tackle specific client group issues. Urban programme funding and other sources of money, such as the European Social Fund, allowed the creation of new projects and community-based services, for example, projects to work with drug abusers or people with HIV-related health problems.

AREA-BASED SERVICES

Most local authority departments are run through the regional or metropolitan tier of local government. The services are grouped into districts and then down to area-based levels. Area-based services serve populations that vary from a few thousand to over 70,000 people. Sparsely populated rural areas obviously require different kinds of service from urban communities. Many area teams, however, have consistent features. These include:

- intake duty systems
- sub-teams based on – communities
  – client specialism
  – the services provided, such as home care or group work.

Most social work departments have organised services to respond to the needs of specific client groups:

- **families and children and young people**
- **elderly and disabled people**
- **offenders (unless they are part of the Probation Service)**
- **people with learning disabilities and mental illness.**

All or most of these forms of service organisation will be represented in area teams or community-based services.

DUTY AND INTAKE SYSTEMS

The solution to accessibility of service has often been the development of teams or groups of staff who are organised within area teams to undertake the first contact work with the public and service users and other agencies who refer cases for the department's attention. Duty officers are available to take phone calls, callers (usually by appointment) and deal with other agencies involved in or referring cases. This contact often represents the first part of assessment.

Different teams have different arrangements for this kind of work. In some teams, all the appropriate staff will be part of a duty rota, but in other teams there will be a specialist group of staff (intake teams) who will deal with all new referrals or short-term work. This could range from simple requests for information and advice, for example, on welfare benefits, or requests for services, such as home help, management of multiple debt when there are threats to cut off essential services or help in dealing with relationship problems that might break up the family.

In one study of the work of an intake team in an English authority (Goldberg et al 1979) there were over 2,000 referrals in one year. The work broke down into several main categories:

- **Disability and Ageing**   30%
- **Financial/Housing**   28%
- **Child/Family**   14%
- **Mental/Emotional**   8%
- **Delinquency**   15%

In urban areas where there are high levels of poverty and deprivation the number of referrals can be much higher and the percentage of referrals about housing and social security issues can also be much higher, perhaps over 50% (Strathclyde Study of Referral Analysis, Freeman & Lambie 1990). Contacts about basic material problems are often the start of complicated child protection and family cases.

Duty systems respond with different types of

involvement to different situations. The receptionist may be able to ensure that a client can get ready access to a required service, such as a bus pass, provided they have the right information. If referrals need more time or home visits are required the duty contact may only involve noting details and making sure the assessed need is passed on to other staff to do fuller assessments or allocate services. Most initial duty or intake appointments or contacts will last between 30-45 minutes. This may seem a short span of time but it has to be seen in the context of other professional contacts. GPs may spend less than 10 minutes with many patients; Balint and Norell (1973) found consultations with GPs lasted 6 minutes on average.

Most social work offices will use standard referral forms to record initial interviews and referrals. This helps staff cover key issues and allows information to be gathered which can be used to compare needs across areas.

Different types of staff are central to an efficient duty and intake response.

- *Reception/Administrative staff* – **apart from the care needed to organise and maintain client-based information systems and information about services, the front line staff who deal with reception duties have to be able to absorb the stress and pressure that many users of social services are carrying as a result of their problems. Every organisation which offers a face-to-face service has to provide a reception facility as its first task (Hall 1974). Clients must be seen on arrival, made welcome, and new arrangements made to make sure they are seen by the right worker from the organisation. This can be difficult work and it is often undervalued by agencies.**

  See Exercise 24.

- *Social Workers* – **qualified workers provide the department's main resource for initial advice and action.**

- *Social Work Assistants/Unqualified Social Workers* – **these staff are often experienced or mature workers with a good working knowledge of welfare systems and the department's role. There would generally be some limitations on the types of cases or work that they would be expected to undertake. It would not be fair to ask untrained staff to assess unsupported the degree or risk in child protection cases or prepare reports for courts.**

34

● ●

EXERCISE 24

What would make a receptionist's job in social services/social work a difficult role? Look at the list below and pick out the things that would worry you about doing the job:

- complicated department
- having to deal with people who are upset
- difficult to find out what people want
- clients may not want to talk about private matters in reception area
- threat of violence from clients.

● ●

Duty and intake teams are usually managed by team leaders or senior social workers and it is their responsibility to run the duty system, check on the quality of the work done, and screen the referrals to decide which deserve priority for future action or services. They also provide cover for the duty staff and act as a resource for advice, consultation and support to them.

The strengths of duty and intake systems are that they allow an early response to be made to people's problems and if the team is well integrated in the communities it serves it can work well with other agencies. Duty and intake work is often about assessment and dealing with emergency or crisis situations. Local knowledge of the community and the informal sources of support for people can be as important as the resources of the agency itself.

On the debit side, the work of the duty and intake team can be determined by 'what comes through the door'. The referrals made by the community itself or other agencies might be more about the problems of poor quality of service response from other departments than social work issues. For example, if social security agencies do not inform people of their rights they turn to social work departments for answers; if housing agencies are not equipped to offer advice then people approach social work departments for help.

When these kinds of problems are presented in volume it makes it more difficult for area teams to tackle statutory work, such as child protection, or tackle long-term work with families or work with communities in developing their own systems of support, like playgroups or advice centres.

Other staff, such as welfare rights officers, managers of domiciliary services, such as home helps, or community development staff, can contribute to the duty and intake team's work.

CHILD CARE

Most studies of social services and social work activity suggest that between ⅔ and ¾ of social workers' time is spent on child care or child-related family work (Social Work Services Group 1992). The range of activities is partly the result of increasing legislation and growing procedural demands on social work staff. It also reflects the complexity of the work and the public and political demand for proper services.

Within an area team there may be 20 or 30 social workers and other kinds of staff working either in specialist sub-teams or patch teams. The bulk of an area team's work here (except probation service) will be with children and young people and families. Further information about this area of work can be found in the *Skills for Caring* books *Families and Groups* and *Protecting Children and Young People.*

The work of social services and social work is partly defined by the law. Most departments will also have key policies that create strategies and objectives for the service. As we outlined in earlier chapters, the policies are shaped by political and moral values as well as economic concerns. The objectives, in turn, identify the most important tasks that staff have to tackle. The work that has to be done and the way it is approached are informed by research and practice experience, drawn from a range of sources including social work, social sciences, medicine and the legal system.

DILEMMAS

Workers may have to take decisions without having a complete understanding of the situation. Care workers often have to come to terms with their own prejudices and feelings as well as the demands of the law and their department's procedures. Two issues, in particular, create strong tensions for care workers – risk management and confidentiality.

Read the 2 examples given then try Exercise 25.

• •

EXERCISE 25

• **Example 1 – What should you do?**
• **Example 2 – How would you respond and what action would you take if the young mother walked out and left you with the baby?**

• •

EXAMPLE 1

Imagine you are a social worker who has been called to a house in the middle of the night by an anonymous phone call, alleging that the children of a nearby family were being abused. When you gain entry to the household you find the parents have been drinking but they are not incapable of looking after the children. The children, aged 5 and 7, are asleep in bed.

The house is untidy but comfortable and there is food in the kitchen. There is no record of the family in the department's files but the couple appear to be in the middle of a serious argument and it turns out that the man has just been made redundant that day. They refuse to disturb the children to allow you to check that they are safe and well. They also say they will not cooperate in the interview until you tell them who 'shopped' them to the department.

EXAMPLE 2

You are a home help with special training to work with HIV/AIDS sufferers. You have been allocated a case where you have to help a young mother take care of a new baby. She is inexperienced in looking after children and lacks confidence in caring for her child. The baby was premature and does not feed or sleep easily. The woman has a history of chronic abuse of drugs and has been involved in prostitution. Since she became pregnant she has been off drugs. It is known that she is HIV positive. Your job is to support her in her role as a mother. When you get to her flat she asks you to look after the baby while she goes out to meet a friend. She offers to pay you money to do this for her and seems to have more cash than usual. She says you're the best worker she's ever had and asks you not to tell anyone about the money.

Care workers have to make judgements like these. They also have to continue offering help to people who don't always want to take it. It should be understood that agencies have structures to support staff to do their jobs. Individual workers may have to take difficult decisions but this should never happen in a vacuum. Apart from training there should be the security of supervision and support from senior staff. The policies and procedures also help to define responses and share the responsibility. Care workers are also part of a team that should be working to a plan – the care plan. In the case scenarios presented there may not be 'right' answers but care workers, with the right support, can often safeguard the welfare of children without displacing the rights of parents.

In recent years, a number of high-profile cases have put social work in the public eye. All care workers have to recognise that their work might be open to this kind of scrutiny as well as the normal supervision and accountability within departments.

The dilemmas faced by staff often centre on the question of risk management. How should statutory departments weigh up the risks of leaving children in the care of parents while there is concern about possible abuse against the damage that will result from taking children away from home? Care workers should be clear about the use and abuse of power but the child's welfare always has to be the first concern.

Confidentiality is an essential element of good care. Unless people are confident about telling care workers significant personal information, and feel that the information will not be abused, then it is difficult to see how problems can be tackled and resources provided. Whenever possible, any sharing of such personal information with other people and agencies should be negotiated with the client. Clients should be asked to give their permission for information to be disclosed. Care workers should not seek or record personal information unless it is relevant to the work being done. Problems start when there is a conflict of interest between clients and other vulnerable people, such as children.

There is a difference between respecting a client's right to privacy and colluding with behaviour which could harm other people. Care workers have to let clients know what information they hold on them and what they will do with the information. They should explain that there is no absolute guarantee of confidentiality. Clients' rights in this area have been legally defined in the **Access to Personal Files Act** 1987 but most

departments will share information and reports as part of good practice. Clients do not have rights to see information about other people. This is often when the difficulties arise for care workers. Our first example described a situation when someone made an allegation about the family. If departments gave out the identity of such callers it would be difficult to encourage people to take action over the abuse of children. Social work agencies need to share information with other agencies, for example, health, police and education.

Children's lives have been lost because professionals felt they should not disclose vital information to each other. Yet again there are no right answers. There can only be the responsible exercise of judgement informed by guidance and support from the agency. (*Skills for Caring – Protecting Children and Young People* will give you help in this area.)

OTHER SOCIAL SERVICE PROVISION

RESIDENTIAL CARE

Many care workers find employment in residential and day care settings. Within most sizeable communities there will be residential children's homes and day care facilities. Accountability for the management of local authority homes and units is sometimes kept within the area team structure, but it is often located with external managers based at district level.

Children's homes have become smaller and more accessible over the years. The trend towards keeping children and young people in the community has meant that the children who do need residential care are often the most vulnerable and damaged in the care system.

The tasks of residential care are shaped by the overall goals for the child care service. Units vary in size between 6-8 beds to more than 23. The work is about personal and physical care and protection of children, married to intervention designed to create change in the lives of the young people in care. To offset the discontinuity (constant staff changes because of shift patterns) of residential life most units have a key worker system. This means that an identified care worker takes responsibility for coordinating aspects of a child's care within the unit and across agencies.

There are the same debates about specialism in residential care as in area teams. Some units act as 'receiving units' building up expertise at helping children and young people when they are taken into care. Others focus on rehabilitation work or help young people learn the skills of independent living when it is clear that returning home is not possible. Increasingly, residential staff are linked into schemes which provide support for young people moving into their own accommodation.

A more controversial area is the establishment of particular units to offer services to children with particular needs, such as disabilities, sexual abuse related problems, or being a member of an ethnic minority. There is always a tension between the belief that all children should be integrated into normal services and the view that some children have a need for special care in separate facilities. Much will depend on local conditions and the availability of resources. In some areas, like island communities, one home may have to serve all these needs.

Local authorities and central government also have to provide residential accommodation for children and young people who have a need for more secure types of care. Throughout the United Kingdom there are facilities for children and young people which tackle this sort of care need. Over the years they have had different titles and functions – Approved Schools, Observation and Assessment Centres, CHE and List 'D' Schools (Scotland). A range of residential schools and special kinds of units, called 'secure accommodation', are in place throughout the country. These are often run by voluntary organisations in cooperation with local authorities.

These young people are often involved in serious crimes or persistently run away but their needs and backgrounds are often identical to other more passive and more obviously vulnerable children. Residential care should offer a refuge – a safe place – for children and young people. It should be a caring response that provides opportunities for control and learning. It should not be cut off from the communities it services, but historical developments of services and lack of cash to provide new resources sometimes mean that children and young people have to live in homes that are some distance from their own families. This makes the chances of keeping in contact with parents more difficult.

The day-to-day challenge of residential care is providing responsive care to meet individual needs and at the same time maintaining control of the behaviour of young people who are often disturbed and distressed.

FOSTER CARE

Foster care is a general term covering temporary care to almost permanent family care, like adoption. Almost 60% of children in care will be placed with foster carers or parents. Agencies recruit and assess foster carers from a wide range of backgrounds but the selection criteria and processes are strict. Although there is evidence of high rates of breakdown of placements it remains a popular option for public care.

Foster carers have had to learn to adapt to the changing needs and requirements of modern social work. Increasingly, departments are recruiting specialist foster carers to deal with particular groups of children. The financial rewards for the work do not adequately reflect the skills and the strain of the role. There are strong pressures, for example, from the National Association of Foster Carers and the British Agencies for Adoption and Fostering, to create a more professional approach to the role of fostering. The trend is towards fee-based schemes rather than basic allowances for the children placed. Fostering is a demanding but worthwhile job. When foster carers are paid fairly and supported by good working relationships with social work staff there is every chance of successful outcomes for vulnerable children. Many foster carers help reunite children with their parents as well as providing substitute family care on a long-term basis.

VOLUNTARY ORGANISATIONS

Most of the large scale voluntary sector organisations, such as churches, Barnardo's, National Children's Homes, Save the Children, the NSPCC and the RSSPCC, and Quarriers, run facilities in all the kinds of settings and family care schemes. They have often been responsible for the introduction of new forms of services, for example, New Families (Barnardos) and Family Centres (NSPCC). They contribute significantly to the resources available for children and young people and their families, and they offer major employment opportunities for care workers.

7

Community care

■ In the recent past, services for elderly and disabled people and their carers were organised through specialist subteams or as part of the workload of generic area teams. They were often simply known as 'elderly' or 'adult' care teams. Adult care teams also dealt with mental health issues and people with learning disabilities.

Since the publication of the White Paper on Community Care, and the introduction of the legislation **(NHS and Community Care Act 1990)** many social services and social work departments have moved towards forming specialist teams that tackle all or some of the client group needs covered by the community care framework.

See Exercise 26.

● ●

EXERCISE 26

In Chapter 1 we outlined the main client groups defined as part of the provision of statutory community care services. How many were there and who were they?

● ●

Community care services are meant to cover:

• **elderly people**
• **dementia sufferers**
• **people with learning disabilities**
• **people with mental illness**
• **people with sensory impairment**
• **people with drug and alcohol related problems**
• **AID/HIV sufferers**
• **people with other progressive illnesses and chronic health problems**
• **all carers.**

Community care reforms will also have an impact on services for children and young people if they have these kinds of problems.

POLICIES AND OBJECTIVES

Many of the values and principles that apply to child care are relevant to all client groups. The brief summary of community care objectives in the panel on page 39 highlights those which reflect the main purpose of the new legislation then, as with the child care section, tries to work out what kinds of tasks care workers take on to achieve the agencies' objectives.

One of the aims of the community care reforms was to pursue better 'value for money' in service provision. The Government believed that this could be achieved by developing a new role for local authorities as an enabling body rather than a monopoly provider of services. This has meant that some departments are transforming themselves into 2 types of work groups – purchasers or providers. This is similar to the changes we looked at in the health services.

Some people consider there are 2 main benefits in organising the services in this way. Firstly, the

COMMUNITY CARE OBJECTIVES

• CARE IN THE COMMUNITY: to identify all people who have need of care and support in the community and to provide the range of services needed to help people remain in their own homes.

• ASSESSMENT: to assess those needs in the context of the individual's situation and involve the clients and their carers in the process.

• INTEGRATION: to enable the integration of elderly and disabled people, and those with mental health problems, into normal domestic and community living. This includes the goal of helping all people in long-term residential, nursing, or hospital care to return to the community, with appropriate support.

• SERVICE DELIVERY AND REVIEW: after assessment of cases and their priority, the arrange of delivery of services to clients and their carers. The delivery of 'packages' of services and care has to be reviewed on a regular basis.

Assessment'. In the official guides to Care Management and Assessment (Dept of Health Social Services Inspectorate and Scottish Office Social Work Services Group 1991) there are 7 key elements to the process. These are:

- **publishing information (about services and resources and agencies)**
- **determining the level of assessment (working out how best to assess need)**
- **assessing need (checking needs against resources and involving clients and carers)**
- **care planning (deciding what's to be done, who's going to do it and how it will be costed and paid for)**
- **implementing the care plan (delivering the services and resources on time and coordinating the work and resources used)**
- **monitoring (checking that the plan is being carried out and that it matches original ideas and costs)**
- **reviewing (making sure that clients/service users, carers and workers sort out whether they think the care plan has worked or needs to be changed).**

Social workers and other care workers based in area teams and specialist teams will deliver many community-based services but the bulk of personal care and direct work with most clients will be carried out by other types of workers in other settings, such as residential units and day care facilities, or by domiciliary (home care) staff. The assessment work is the link between a client's and his carer's needs and access to the required resources. One of the biggest problems in social care is how to get the right services to the right people at the right time. All care systems have to involve clients and carers in making the right decisions about assessed needs and care plans.

The first decision to be made is who is responsible for pulling the assessment and care management work together. This can depend on a number of factors, including the complexity of the case and the degree of specialist knowledge required to understand the problems and needs of particular client groups. Generally, assessment will be the responsibility of promoted, qualified or trained staff.

Other care workers have a contribution to make to the assessment and service delivery. To illustrate some of the roles and work involved we will consider some different client groups and how services are organised to respond to their particular needs.

managers and care workers who assess the needs and hold the budget, the purchasers, have a vested interest in getting the most for their clients out of the money they hold on their behalf. It is argued that these managers and care workers will be able to look after the interests of clients and users more effectively because they are not responsible for running the services that are used.

Secondly, the split encourages other providers (particularly the private and voluntary sector) to bid to provide services. In this approach, the local authority might deliver services to clients as well as arranging service delivery, but the local authority services would have to compete with other providers for the available funds and budget. From April 1993, local authorities will receive the social security payments paid to individuals for residential and nursing care. This will be a large part of the funding for community care. However, many agencies still operate along more traditional lines.

The method of organising services and work related to community care client groups has come to be described as 'Care Management and

---

ELDERLY CARE

Read the Example in the panel then try Exercise 27.

EXAMPLE

Mr Thomas is 83 years old and lives alone in a small mining village. His wife died last year. She managed all the household work and did the cooking for them both. Although they had a large family only one daughter, Nancy, and her family live nearby. Nancy is a lone parent and has to work full time. She usually visits her Dad in the evenings.

Mr Thomas has arthritis and a heart condition. Since his wife's death his physical and emotional health has been poor. He is virtually helpless in the house. As an ex-miner he gets 'free' coal and kept a coal-fired system for heating and hot water when his house was renovated by the council. Nancy's GP phoned the social services department to see if the family could get some support because Nancy was becoming stressed and exhausted by the level of care her Dad needed.

● ●

EXERCISE 27

On the basis of the information given in the Example who should be involved in assessing Mr Thomas's and Nancy's needs? What are their needs going to be and what kind of services would be likely to help the family and be acceptable to them?

● ●

Did the GP discuss his suggestion to refer the family to social services with Mr Thomas and Nancy? It would be difficult to take the assessment forward without the family's cooperation. Ideally, Mr Thomas and Nancy should be at the heart of the assessment.

This kind of case might well be allocated to a qualified social worker but it could be handled by an experienced social work assistant. Some teams might judge that the referral should be taken on by the staff most likely to be involved in the long-term management of the case. In Mr Thomas's situation this could be the domiciliary or home care staff. Visits to the family homes and discussions with the family, GP and district nurse might be enough to build up a good initial picture of Mr Thomas's circumstances and Nancy's position. It takes skill to negotiate the level of trust needed to explore honestly the needs that Mr Thomas has, and it has to be done within a reasonable period of time to be relevant to the family's concerns.

A list of needs and objectives for dealing with their needs might be:

- *Personal and physical care:* **Mr Thomas needs help with setting and keeping his coal fire going, cooking and mobility.**
- *Social contact:* **Mr Thomas needs to increase his level of social contact.**
- *Money:* **Mr Thomas needs help to manage his affairs and apply for the benefits to which he and Nancy are entitled. There are no debts at present but he has used his savings to get by.**
- *Grief:* **Mr Thomas has only started to acknowledge the death of his wife. His grief has robbed him of much of his will to deal with his practical problems.**
- *Support for carer:* **Nancy is on the verge of physical and mental collapse. She needs to know that she is not Mr Thomas's only source of support. If Nancy can see that other kinds of help are available on a planned basis she can allow herself to spend time on her own personal and family needs.**

KEY SERVICE AND THE CARE WORKER

Most of the care workers, including the GP and the district nurse, could argue that they play the key role in Mr Thomas's case. In terms of time Nancy is the main carer but each of the professional workers and the informal carers all play their part. The important question to address is which service will make the difference between Mr Thomas managing to stay in the community or having to move into other forms of care?

The key to Mr Thomas's ability to carry on living in his own home is the Home Help Service (Home Care). Originally, this service was run by health authorities as a support to mothers during confinement. Over the years it moved from health to welfare and is now associated much more with elderly care. About 90% of home help clients will be elderly people. The service, however, does reach across all client groups. It is usually allocated for a period of about 2 hours for a number of days a week. Charges are normally made but are often nominal or waived when people have very low incomes. Home helps often work part time and they represent some of the largest staff groups in local authority departments. They are paid nationally agreed salary levels and have begun to attract additional responsibilities and training opportunities that reflect the social and personal care elements of their work.

The home help service is labour intensive and costly to provide. Although the value of the service in terms of user response is recognised, many authorities have made moves towards contracting out domiciliary care to private and voluntary organisations.

The home help/care service can provide both personal care and practical assistance that can really make a difference to people's lives (see *Skills for Caring – Home Care Services*).

DAY SERVICES

As their name suggests, day services are run on a different basis from residential care. Day care means that clients don't have to leave their own home or community. The value of day care is in the flexibility and positive contribution it provides to help people stay in their own homes. Day care also provides relief and respite for carers. When carers have a clear block of time to rest and meet their own needs – and are confident that someone else will be providing a good quality of care to their partner, relative or friend – even high levels of dependency can be manageable. The range of day care facilities for all client groups is wide. At the informal end of the range there are lunch clubs and social activities. These services offer company and can be used to make sure basic physical needs are being met, for example, lunch clubs. At the other end, entry to the resource can be strictly controlled and the work of the centre or unit can be tightly focused to achieve defined goals, for example, rehabilitation groups for stroke victims.

Day services can also act as a link between clients and other systems. Some agencies see day care services as transitional – a place to go to prepare for the future or a place to go to ease a return into the wider society. For instance, in a day care resource centre the activities are organised to suit a varied set of users and clients. If there are clients with severe disabilities then resources like health care and speech therapy will come to the centre.

CARE PLAN FOR MR THOMAS

Mr Thomas's situation has positive elements. He has insight into his difficulties. He loves Nancy and her children and he appreciates her care of him and her need for support in the task. He wants to stay in his own home.

The home care organiser goes to meet Nancy and Mr Thomas some weeks later and proposes the following arrangements for care:

• A home help will visit daily to prepare breakfast and start Mr Thomas's fire and do his shopping. She will return at lunchtime to make Mr Thomas a snack. Over time, and depending on Mr Thomas's health and confidence, the home help will work with Mr Thomas in developing some basic cooking skills.

• An occupational therapist will call to assess Mr Thomas's capacity for movement and also to check on aids and adaptations for the house. The occupational therapist will work with Mr Thomas for a limited period.

• A social worker with experience of bereavement work with elderly people will visit Mr Thomas to help him deal with his grief.

• Local organisations, including Mrs Thomas's old church, have been approached to involve Mr Thomas in social events and volunteer visiting.

• A period of respite care on a 24-hour basis has been organised for 2 months ahead to give Nancy a holiday and she will be given financial assistance for this.

The home care organiser will meet with Nancy, Mr Thomas and the district nurse to review how the plan is working in 6 weeks time. The review will involve health-based staff since their involvement has to be fitted into the package of care and they referred the case in the first instance. What might emerge from the review is an update of the diary of care and support that ensures Mr Thomas is well supported and that there is no duplication of effort in providing services.

With other clients, the focus is on linking them to normal services, such as education, leisure and recreation. Others are involved in preparation for employment. Each client has a detailed schedule of goals and achievements to guide their activity and the work of the staff with them. Assessment tools and programmes have been developed to bring out the best in the clients.

For children, day care can be nurseries, preschool and early years provision. For the elderly, the service can be lunch clubs, drop-in centres, or intensive support based in residential complexes. For adults, day care can be provided for almost any client group, such as people with disabilities and health problems, addiction-related problems, offenders and mentally ill people.

The staff in day care come from different backgrounds. The qualified staff can be trained in social work, teachers, occupational therapists or health-trained professionals. Many projects work on multidisciplinary lines. Innovative projects sometimes start off as day care and end up as small businesses providing employment for the users. Local authorities and voluntary organisations employ people with different backgrounds and skills to work as instructors and care staff in day care services. There are often drivers working for the centres to meet transport needs and domestic staff can also become involved in programmes and in working with the clients.

COMMUNITY CARE DILEMMAS

We saw that, in child care, working with community care client groups presents risks and anxieties; working in residential care and day care adds other pressures.

INDIVIDUALITY

The essence of good caring is respect for people as individuals. In both group care and group living the needs of individuals are potentially at odds with the group. Treating people individually takes time. Most establishments have staffing based on a staff:client ratio. In almost all care settings – health, education and social work – careful planning is needed to make sure people get enough individual attention, without undermining their independence.

The pressures on care workers can lead to insensitivity and the features of institutional care that depress staff and clients alike. If clients are 'batched and processed' for routine bathing, toileting and feeding then personal care has been replaced by impersonal care. Individuality is bound up with space and resources. Having a room to yourself by choice is valued personal space. This does not mean that everything that involves group processes works against individual care. A good meal shared with other people can be a fulfilling social encounter. Eating a cold meal off plastic plates, in silence at a table with people you don't like and at a time that suits the shift pattern of the home, might not be the highlight of your day.

Good care is marked by the care workers' ability to promote genuine choices by clients in everyday living and by responding to people as individuals. The challenge for the care worker is the management of the group's 'life space' and the resources of the unit – especially their own time – to create personal care.

CHOICE AND RISK MANAGEMENT

Creating choice is part of the care worker's job. The more personal an issue is, the more choice matters. All adults should be free to make choices, as long as their choices don't conflict with other people's choices and well-being. Making rules and regulations in residential homes is an attempt to get round this problem. However, rules themselves generate other difficulties – they put staff in positions of power and control that limit the potential for good care.

Another dilemma care workers face is what to do if the choices offered involve risk. For example:

- **In a day care unit for confused clients should the door be kept locked?**
- **If there are fire regulations to be upheld should care workers stop someone leaving doors open or deter smoking in bed?**
- **If a hostel for people with a drink problem has a policy of 'no alcohol' should residents be allowed to drink?**

Group living and care throw up these conflicts every day. Agencies have to observe regulations, for example, in health and safety legislation, and codes set down in law for care standards. Managers and care workers in homes and centres do not have discretion in all areas of the establishment's regime.

Sometimes the price of independence and client choice will be physical harm. Care workers have to balance out what both the long-term and the immediate consequences of their style of care will be. If an elderly resident is not allowed to practise keeping control of his bladder and toileting himself the end result will be dependency on staff to help him. It may seem easier in the short run to use incontinence pads rather than spend time helping someone regain control of their own bodily functions, but how do you measure the shame of wetting yourself and sitting in your own urine against the pain and effort of getting to the toilet in time and publicly displaying your struggle?

The problem for care workers in this kind of situation is partly rooted in the quality of understanding and communication between them and their clients. If clients cannot articulate clearly what they want it is difficult to do the right thing. Continuity of relationships and patience are often the best resources care workers have to get to know what clients want. When the key worker model works well there is a basic building block for such understanding. Standards of care and ideas about what 'good' care is vary with the values and beliefs of people.

We have already drawn attention to the fact that no one care worker or agency has a monopoly on care – it is a shared responsibility which should have the client in the middle. Relatives and carers can present care workers with insoluble problems if they want different outcomes of care and different types of care for the client. Homes and units have to work hard to get agreement about the way they work in these situations. When relatives 'put' a client in a home (as they see it) there can be strong feelings about the process. Many complaints will be justified, but there will be other occasions when what is being rehearsed are unresolved feelings about rejecting the client. Hard working staff can find reproaches about lack of care hurtful if there seems to be no basis for the complaints. The involvement of carers in assessing and planning care can help defuse these tensions. There has to be a balance between the rights of clients, their carers, and the workers involved.

RIGHTS

Residents in care are by definition vulnerable people. It is unusual for them to have chosen to be in care. In some cases they may have been required to accept care and supervision, for example, Mental Health legislation gives local authorities powers to put people in hospital care or determine where they should live. In other cases, physical debility can undermine clients' abilities to exercise their rights.

It is important that care workers remember to consider the rights of residents and that they help them exercise these rights. Clients are citizens, that is, able to vote and use legal systems and entitled to benefits, health care, and access to all normal services. One of the goals of care should be the fullest expression of citizenship and the culture of the unit is the place to start to reinforce this. If clients are not involved in decisions that affect them, do not have access to information held about them, or are not able to have contact with people outside the unit (phone, letters, visitors and visits) it is unlikely that they will feel like citizens. The longer the period that clients have to remain in care in any setting the more important it is that they have a say in how the place is run. Maintaining high levels of client participation can be hard work and is often resented by more insecure care workers and managers who feel threatened by what they see as the possibility of anarchy. If there are splits within the staff group about levels of client autonomy there can be considerable tension in a unit. Clear leadership and staff participation are needed to nurture client independence. Care workers cannot help clients maintain self-respect unless they feel their own contribution is valued. (This topic is developed further in *Skills for Caring – Families and Groups*.)

8

Services for offenders

BACKGROUND ISSUES

The other main client group that attracts statutory services is offenders. Offenders are a minority client group compared to elderly people or children and families but, despite this, crime is a major source of political and moral controversy. Crime is costly: victims and property bear the costs in human and financial terms; offenders and their families suffer the consequences of punishment, society has to pay for retribution – reprisal in the shape of punishment – and prisons and other types of care and treatment are expensive.

Although there are marked differences between England and Wales, Northern Ireland, and Scotland, in the way services are provided for offenders and the different legal systems, the government has decided on national objectives for offender work. The objectives have been defined by national standards and priorities and funding to local authorities and the probation service has been tied to performance in meeting these goals. In effect, this means that all offender services are contracted out by the government. The money paid to the probation service and local authority social work departments (in Scotland) depends on the results provided by the services.

This control of the use of funding and the priorities of the service providers has developed over the past few years. Although criminal justice legislation has always defined the main activities of the services for offenders and court-related work, the radical changes outlined have been brought about by government decisions and negotiation rather than changes in the law. The new 'National Objectives' (and the Standards, or Priorities, applied in Scotland, England and Wales) do not have a statutory basis. The supply of money controls the response by the services.

The performance of the services is monitored by setting targets for the quantity of results achieved, for example, reduction of custody (prison) disposals or number of visits made, and the quality of service provided, for example, the length of time taken to provide reports and the standard achieved.

We have already noted some of the differences between Scotland and the rest of the United Kingdom in services and organisation. In Scotland, all statutory social work services to offenders are provided by local authority social work departments. In the rest of the United Kingdom the services are provided largely by a separate probation service. The probation service is linked directly to the Home and Health Department in central government, and run by Chief Probation Officers on a regional level. Area Probation Teams provide the direct services and are accountable to the Chief Probation Officer. Local Probation Committees draw together relevant bodies to influence the delivery of services and cooperation at a local level.

POLICY AND SERVICE OBJECTIVES

There are 4 broad objectives in the national framework and these are shown in the panel.

AGENCY SERVICES AND WORKER ACTIVITIES

Resources are allocated to agencies on the basis of expected workload. Specialist teams or social workers (or a proportion of the time of social workers) provide services in the area teams and communities. In addition, specialist teams and staff are located in key settings for offenders. These are

POLICY OBJECTIVES

1. REDUCING THE LEVEL OF CUSTODY
To reduce the use of custody (prison or other forms of detention) whether for remand (awaiting trial) or as a sentence of the court (punishment). The achievement of this goal depends on the availability of suitable community-based alternatives.

2. DEVELOPMENT OF 'THROUGH CARE' SERVICES
To provide a proper continuity of service and care at all stages of the offender's involvement in the criminal justice system – at court when being sentenced, in prison, on release, and in the community.

3. TACKLING OFFENDER BEHAVIOUR
To help offenders tackle their offending behaviour, and assist them to live socially responsible lives within the law.

4. FAMILY SUPPORT
To assist the families and carers of offenders where the family life suffers because of the offending behaviour.

prisons, courts, state hospitals, probation hostels and centres. Much of the work has to be undertaken by qualified social workers or probation officers, but there are other types of care workers involved with offenders – assistants, supervisors and instructors, as well as residential and day care staff.

ASSESSMENT

The key to work with offenders, as with other client groups, is assessment. Assessment is essential if care workers and other agencies want to know what and how to tackle the offender's needs and concerns. The added responsibility in offender work is that courts want to have advice about how they should deal with offenders. The reports for the court are called Social Enquiry Reports or Social Background Reports (sometimes called SERs or SBRs as a shorthand name). The reports are intended to help the sentencing of offenders by giving the court reliable information and analysis of the offender's personality and social

circumstances, as they relate to his or her offending.

The probation officer or social worker can also make suggestions to the court about what kind of sentence would work best or what the likely impact of a particular disposal would be. The court usually wants to know what the offender's attitude is to the offence. The court takes account of the report and other factors when sentencing. Except in very serious cases, the court reports are only prepared after the offender has been found guilty or pled guilty to the offence or offences.

The report should be the basis of the care plan for the offender. The action required of services and the offender should be negotiated and presented to the court at the time of sentencing. The probation department or social work department will have their own mechanisms for case review but the court can also be used to assess progress. A number of disposals build scope for reappearing at court into the sentence.

PREPARING A REPORT

The offender is interviewed by the social worker (probably more than once) and family members and other interested parties are seen or contacted. Confirmation of statements might be sought by reports from other sources, for example, doctors or schools, and the records of agencies. The reports are usually prepared using a structured schedule or agenda, or a list of areas that have to be investigated and considered. This helps provide the courts with a reasonable standard of reports and some consistency in their style. Part of the report focuses on the risk of reoffending and an assessment of the offender's 'criminal career' – what, why, and when.

Although there will be interest in the offender's biography and personal history, most reports tend to concentrate on the recent past and current situation in the offender's life. The department may already know the offender from previous work. Most departments ensure that the worker responsible for a case, or best known to the client, is allocated any new work in relation to that client. This is part of the continuity of care that should be given.

The offender should have an opportunity to go over the possible sentencing options that are likely and express his or her views about them; the cooperation given should be included in the report. Occasionally, a worker may have to go to court to speak to the report.

ALTERNATIVES TO CUSTODY

This is the main reason for the government's financial support of social work for offenders. The prison population in the United Kingdom is high relative to most European countries. Conditions in many prisons are unacceptable. Prison riots and roof top protests are embarrassing to a government. Unless the numbers can be contained and reduced then the only option is an increase in the prison building programme. On the grounds of humanity and economic costs prisons are not always the answer. Probation officers and social workers can help prevent custody in a number of ways.

Reports

The assessment work undertaken during preparation of reports is preventive. Reports are requested on the basis of the age and vulnerability of offenders, and the risk of imprisonment. Reports include information on physical and mental health (psychiatric illness is common among offenders in the prison population), on drug problems, and on the risk of self-injury or suicide. Judges often adjourn, that is, take a break or postpone, the court proceedings to ask probation officers or social workers based at court to talk to offenders before deciding on what to do with them. If the court needs more information, for example, a psychiatric report, it might want the offender to attend court in a few weeks. The judge will want to be certain the offender will reappear. One sure way to have the offender turn up is remanding the offender. This means the offender is held in custody until the new court date. This puts pressure on the prison system.

The probation officer or social worker may be able to advise the judge about the risk of bail or if there are bail hostels or other alternatives to custody. These activities all happen before the final sentence is passed.

Fines

Many offenders are fined by courts and fail to pay. Eventually, they end up in prison for nonpayment. Probation and social work departments can offer supervision of fine payments in conjunction with court officials. They also provide welfare rights and debt management advice to make sure vulnerable offenders and families get their benefit entitlement sorted out. This helps payment and cuts down imprisonment.

The main preventive work of the departments is to offer the courts realistic alternatives to custody, such as sentencing options and proper after care to stop reoffending. The court disposals that are used as alternatives to custody include probation orders and community service orders.

Probation

Probation means supervision in the community by a probation officer or social worker. All probation orders have legal requirements, including that the offender:

- **must be 'of good behaviour' and not offend**
- **conform to the directions of the supervising officer**
- **let the officer know of any change in address or employment.**

Additional requirements can be added, such as paying back compensation for the crime or attending for psychiatric treatment. Probation can also be linked to a residential requirement, like a probation hostel, or attending special programmes, such as one for sex offenders.

Orders last from 6 months to 3 years. If offenders don't respond and commit further offences then the supervising officer can take the matter back to court (breach of probation) and have the judge reconsider the case. There are guidelines about the level of contact and supervision of probationers.

More than any other kind of disposal from the court the probation order relies on the relationship skills of the supervising officer to confront and effect change in the offender's life. The work lends itself to group work approaches. Probation and social work departments are charged with the duty of providing offenders with 'advice, guidance, and assistance'. This duty has not changed greatly from the original court missionaries at the turn of the century. The models and techniques used have developed but the heart of the process depends on a good 'helping relationship'.

Comunity service

These orders differ from probation in that they are clearly a penalty. They are meant to give the court an alternative when custody would be almost inevitable. Supervision during community service is not meant to be treatment or casework. It should focus on the task of ensuring the offender complies with the order – turns up on time and does the work properly. The offender is sentenced to do unpaid work in the community to pay for the crime. The penalty is imposed for a specified number of hours and suitability for community service is assessed.

The schemes are run by probation and social

work departments and they have to provide a range of constructive and challenging work placements for the courts to consider and use. The work should not be demeaning or unrealistic for any offender. At its best, the work releases undeveloped talents and provides basic experience which is converted into training and new careers. Many offenders discover abilities they didn't know they had. If the order is breached then the supervising officer can ask to review the order and the original custodial sentence might then be considered.

Placements are organised in a variety of settings including care establishments.

Through care

During prison sentences offenders can have access to support programmes provided by prison-based social workers or probation officers. These staff also form a link between prison and community-based services. Offenders should be allocated a supervising officer for parole or after care (depending on the length of the sentence) before release from prison. The work to plan their reintegration in society should have been well under way before they leave. The level of practical support required can be extensive – money, accommodation and employment all present problems to many offenders leaving custody. For prisoners who have spent long terms in custody the adjustment for themselves and their families can be traumatic.

Read the Example on the right then try Exercise 28.

• •

EXERCISE 28

Given Tam's background what do you think you will recommend to the court and how will you justify what you suggest?

• •

When the assessment is made for court, the judge or magistrate wants to know a great deal about the background of the offender and the pattern of previous offending behaviour. In Tam's case almost all his criminal activity was carried out with a known group of young men in his old neighbourhood. Tam has moved from there and has the chance of a new start. He cares for his girlfriend and although he is anxious about being a father he is very excited about the prospect. He has put a lot of effort into making their new home comfortable and has done all the work himself. His girlfriend has had to give up work and he knows he

> **EXAMPLE**
>
> Let us find out what you would make of Tam's situation as the social worker who has been asked to submit a report to the court about him. Tam is large and angry – he is out in the office waiting room. You have asked him to meet you in the office to discuss the preparation of the court report. The receptionist had a hard time getting him to calm down and take a seat.
>
> You know little about him from personal contact since his case has been transferred from another area. He is presently on after-care supervision. In the last office where his case was held there was no one to take on the work and he called for 'duty' appointments to meet the conditions of the after-care supervision.
>
> Tam is 23 and he and his girlfriend were allocated a house in the local estate. She is 19 and pregnant. He has a background of serious assaults and thefts. The present charge relates to an offence against a neighbour in the new area. Tam alleges the man was abusive to his girlfriend and he 'sorted him out'. The man required hospital care.
>
> In the interview that follows you discover that Tam's history of offending has a number of features that suggest he presents a high risk of getting into further trouble. These include: a lot of previous convictions spread evenly over time; he was very young when he first got into trouble; he has been in residential care or custody almost every year since he was 10; and it is only 6 months since he was released from his last prison sentence.

has to find work to keep them. He has made real efforts to find work.

Tam has had no support from the department since his release and got his house by himself. He resents this charge. He cannot promise he would not do the same again but accepts that he probably over-reacted to the situation. It was a different sort of offence from his past crimes – no alcohol or other people were involved, and there was no theft.

47

Tam felt it was right that he took action to defend his wife.

Part of what the court needs to know is whether any risks that can be taken are reasonable. Has Tam reached a turning point in his life? What if the department made a commitment to help Tam, how would he respond? This last point is crucial in determining if probation could work. If the social worker and the offender believe that the relationship can be used to change the situation then the report to the court can start with that commitment.

This was a real case that turned out well for Tam and his new family. It could easily have ended up with a broken relationship, a lone parent existence for his girlfriend, and Tam a more hardened criminal. Tam was placed on probation.

THE VOLUNTARY SECTOR

There are a number of voluntary organisations that act to promote the welfare of offenders and provide services for them. The **National Association for the Care and Resettlement of Offenders** (**NACRO** and in Scotland, **SACRO**) provides support for offenders and runs hostels and other projects. **APEX** is an organisation concerned with employment and training for offenders. A range of employment opportunities exist in these caring agencies.

Victim Support is a national concern supported by monies from central government and local authorities. Volunteer counsellors visit victims of crime and offer emotional support and practical help.

The national objectives require departments to plan their services in conjunction with voluntary organisations.

DILEMMAS AND CONCERNS

WELFARE AND JUSTICE

The tension between care and control is evident throughout work with offenders. Social workers and probation officers are officers of the court; their first duty is to the court and in that role they are part of the criminal justice system. They often work side by side with the police and the prison service dealing with the same clients. Society tends to see probation and community service as soft options but the offenders can find the system quite intrusive and painful. The main tasks of the police and prison system are deterring, catching and containing offenders. The key role of the welfare services is helping offenders reform and keeping people out of custody. The objectives of the agencies do not always sit well together.

The law assumes that people take responsibility for their own actions. The welfare model explains behaviour as the result of social pressures as well as personal choice. Different agencies see offenders in different ways. Offenders find their way into the system by a variety of routes but poverty, homelessness, psychiatric illness and racial discrimination are often part of the process. Probation officers and social workers have to acknowledge these factors and represent them in the system.

The area of risk management in offender work is stark. If workers make the wrong decisions the consequences can be serious. If dangerous offenders are placed in the community and do not respond to the planned service offered then the community can suffer.

PRIORITIES

One of the reasons that the Scottish system for working with offenders was redefined by the national framework was the pressure that came from other areas of work. Child care issues tended to predominate. The 100% funding of offender work meant the government could expect priority for offenders.

This had been one of the main arguments for retaining the probation service elsewhere.

YOUNG PEOPLE IN TROUBLE

All 3 systems (in Scotland, England and Wales, and Northern Ireland) have different age bands and approaches for dealing with young people in trouble. Even in Scotland, where the Children's Hearings system can keep young people in the care system until they are 18, the tendency is to let go early. Once young people are in the criminal justice arena they move into more serious forms of control rapidly – particularly young girls.

The **Children Act 1989** will provide more scope for the prevention of the criminalisation of young people but there is still a need to hold onto them beyond the age of 16. At present, funding falls between the 2 stools of 'child care' and 'offenders'. The right kinds of services are not in place to respond to youth homelessness, drug abuse and runaways.

9

The caring services in the nineties

■ The only thing we can be certain about in the 1990s is constant change. The political and ideological shifts of the 1980s have been confirmed but the precise shape of services has yet to evolve. Local government will be reformed. Community care will become 'business' in earnest as the money moves from social security to local authorities in 1993. The health service will experience 'opting out' on a greater scale. 'Europe 1992' will become a reality. The pace of change has accelerated and it is unlikely to slow down. Care workers in the services have to come to terms with change and those entering the services have to recognise the impact such changes will have on their working lives.

In the final chapter of the book we will examine some of the important themes of change and define what they will mean for the caring services and clients.

ACCOUNTABILITY

The government-led reform of public sector care has several key objectives, these are the:

- **development of competition in all areas of service provision, partly by separating purchasing from providing services**
- **expansion of private sector providers in social care services**
- **control of public expenditure (the money the government spends)**
- **use of value for money techniques to evaluate services and their quality**
- **shift of control of services away from large bureaucracies and political bodies (like local authorities) towards independent agencies under the direction of professional managers**

- **effective coordination and planning of services across all agencies.**

At the same time, there has been a crisis of confidence in many areas of the public sector services. Child care and community care services have been criticised heavily in public inquiries and investigations. There has been constant argument about the cost of public care and the Audit Commission has been used to highlight alleged waste and inefficiency.

The direct consequences of these developments can be seen in the changing shape of the number and types of agencies competing to provide services and secure resources. The government has recognised the twin problems of unregulated care services and the need to monitor the performance of the public sector. The strategy it has promoted to deal with these concerns has 3 parts:

- **They will control who gets public money and watch how it is spent.**
- **The consumer will be given a voice and encouraged to use it.**
- **The activities of care providers will be subject to scrutiny by outsiders.**

Much of this strategy is laid out in the government's Citizen's Charter. There will be detailed charters for each major area of service in the public sector. The essential features of the 'watchdog' system include:

- Planning
- Inspection and audit
- Complaints
- Access to personal information
- Quality assurance
- Training

49

PLANNING

All areas of the health and social work services have to be provided on a planned basis. This obligation is defined in law for community care. The plans must be public documents and contain detailed information about services. This information has to deal with targets and standards for the development of care. There must be consultation with all interested parties and the health and social work services have to work to plan their services jointly with the other providers of related services. There has to be mechanism to review the plans. Plans in this form will help empower client groups and communities and allow the government to hold services to the goals they have set and agreed.

INSPECTION AND AUDIT

The **NHS and Community Care Act 1990** required local authorities to set up independent 'arms length' inspection units. These will inspect all community care and child care units and services that are registered to provide care. Annual reports which are public documents will be made available. Inspection units will have a powerful role in setting standards of care and making agencies live up to them. In both England and Wales, and recently in Scotland, an equivalent inspectorate responding to a national focus has been established.

The Audit Commission and its Scottish equivalent are busy working on a programme of evaluation of public sector performance. Their past work did much to underpin the reforms of community care provision. In time, their reports on individual authorities will probably become accessible to the public and be used to challenge poor management. It is likely that league tables will be constructed that allow comparison between authorities.

These scrutiny developments can, and will, have an impact on individual care workers and work places but they will focus on the 'big' agenda of service planning and expenditure. Other proposals will have a more direct effect on care workers and establishments.

COMPLAINTS

The community care legislation has introduced a formal complaints system in the public sector for clients and their carers. This extends to other client groups as well as community care. The system lays down requirements about how complaints and representations must be handled. Active representation and support for people making complaints will be encouraged. Most voluntary organisations and private concerns will find that they also need to have a complaints machinery to get funding or business. The handling of complaints will be an important part of how services are assessed.

ACCESS TO PERSONAL INFORMATION

Starting with social work in 1987, all the main services in the public sector have had legislation passed which entitles people to see what personal information agencies hold about them. Coupled with the complaints machinery this allows clients to find out a great deal more about services they have received.

QUALITY ASSURANCE

The White Paper, *Care in the Community* (HMSO 1989) set itself the goal of developing a flourishing independent service alongside good quality public care. It is too soon to judge how effective the reforms will be. The pursuit of quality is difficult to argue against; much of the Citizen's Charter initiative is based on quality assurance. This management philosophy has been taken from manufacturing and industrial models of management and applied to the social care field. Critics argue that clients are not consumers because they don't have choice and neither are their problems mechanical nor their needs simple. What *is* certain is that the notion of quality assurance is in vogue and care workers can expect to find that defining and assessing quality will be a management priority in the 1990s. In agencies with a healthy and participative style clients and care workers will get a chance to define the standards that are achievable and important.

TRAINING

One of the main challenges of the 1990s will be the creation of a well-trained work force in social and health care. The significance of training for care workers cannot be over-emphasised. Every day, approximately 500,000 care workers carry out the tasks of caring. The great majority of them carry out this work without the benefit of adequate training. The limited training that some obtain is not recognised formally. Worst of all, the majority do not achieve any recognition that the skills and knowledge they use every day display competence. This has created a sense of division in social care between qualified and unqualified staff. Career prospects and conditions of pay have tended to be based on the achievement of a narrow range of qualifications which are not accessible to the majority of care workers. Personal qualities are essential to begin a good carer but training is also needed to get the best out of people.

The development of vocational training is well under way. Health and social care qualifications are planned that will create new opportunities for care workers. Unlike the older models, **National Vocational Qualifications (NVQs)** and **Scottish Vocational Qualifications (SVQs)** will be progressive and eventually integrate with other levels of training and qualification. The full range of NVQs will take time to emerge but achievement will count towards higher levels and care workers will be able to achieve results by demonstrating competence through assessment by their ordinary work as well as studying on courses. Training affirms competence and creates confidence. Care workers need to know they can take on the role that society requires of them.

Competencies are based on the application of knowledge, attitudes and skills. Increasingly, agencies and educators are recognising that the core competencies required by different settings are consistent – training is becoming a multidisciplinary process. This was recognised over a decade ago by the Jay (1979) and Warnock (1978) reports. Just as agencies are finally learning to work with each other, the planning of education and training is beginning to reflect a full partnership between employers and educational establishments.

There will still be the need for specialist training for professional groups, for example, probation officers or health visitors, but this can be met through focused training designed to develop skills and learning, for example, post qualification training and areas of particular practice in the Diploma in Social Work. When the roles and the tasks converge the training lends itself to a joint approach, with staff from different backgrounds coming together to learn from each other as much as from the formal teaching, as in the Diploma in Community Care.

The rate of funding and targets for the number of trained staff will be important measures of the government's willingness to resource health and social care. All care workers can contribute to this goal by asserting their need for training within agencies. The dignity of care given to clients is strengthened by the self-respect that training can offer care workers.

REPRESENTATION BY CARE WORKERS

There have been 2 models of organisation for care workers and professional staff. One involves the use of organised labour through trades unions and the other is the professional organisation or association, like the British Medical Association (BMA). In health occupational groups there has been a tendency to combine both, creating a significant power base. Registration for membership in General Councils has been the medical model and such Councils and related bodies for doctors, nurses, midwives and health visitors carry responsibilities for serious questions of discipline as well as insurance and negotiating rights.

This leaves out a vast army of ancillary staff in health care who usually join a main public sector union, such as **UNISON**, the **Public Service Union**, or the **General and Municipal Workers Union (GMWU)**. Social work and social care have professional organisations, the **British Association of Social Workers (BASW)** and the **Social Care Association (SCA),** but they do not normally act as negotiating parties with employers and they do not have disciplinary powers that can affect the ability to practise. These issues are left to employers and unions.

The government's reforms have been started largely without the cooperation of trades unions. The emergence of the independent sector and private competition has eroded trade union influence over service delivery and planning. Value-for-money exercises and competition have often meant a reduction in wages for care workers and pressure to work in nonunion organisations.

Consultation with the professional associations also had a similar lack of impact on the pace and shape of reforms. In political terms it is hard for organised groups of staff to convince the wider audience that their interests are always convergent with those of clients.

In his study for the National Institute of Social Work, Parker (1990) advocates a strong case for a register of social workers and social care staff. This is seen as one way of regulating poor practice and misconduct by practitioners and providing a coherent voice to deal with media and political criticism of the caring agencies. It seems likely that some new organisations will emerge to represent workers in social work and social care.

of people on the basis of race and gender will throw up a similar conflict between the values of trained care workers and the policies and practices of the caring agencies and the other parts of the welfare system.

ANTIOPPRESSIVE WORKING

Technical skills and knowledge can be developed through access to training. A much harder kind of learning has to be encountered to sort out the value base of individual care workers and their agencies. In many programmes of training, the requirements have moved beyond awareness to a positive demonstration of ability to 'understand and counteract the impact of stigma and discrimination on grounds of poverty, age, disability and sectarianism' (CCETSW Paper 30 Dip SW, 1991); and to combat individual and institutional racism through anti-racist practice. Gender issues and sexism also have to be confronted.

Care workers have to witness the reality and the results of oppression based on race, class and gender. Just as police officers cannot walk away from trouble on the streets so care workers have to confront the issues directly in their working environment. Achieving status as trained or qualified workers will involve the assessment of performance in this area as much as any other skill or task.

The integrity of good care will depend on care workers' honesty and moral courage as much as on the development of the policies of agencies. Britain is a complex multicultural society and discrimination will continue to pose a threat to justice and the quality of services. Care workers probably have to start with their own agencies – gender and race issues abound in the caring services as much as any other form of organisation. There are inherent tensions in belonging to a professional group which requires sound values and attitudes of its workers but tends not to tackle the oppression within its own systems.

During the 1970s, the political tensions in social work were expressed in the dilemma of working with individuals when wider societal change and justice was needed. Work with individuals was seen 'as papering over the cracks' of an inadequate welfare state. Community work and social change were advocated as the priority. This led to conflict between workers and their agencies and between social services and other agencies. Unless positive action is taken on a dramatic scale the oppression

CONCLUSION

We have tried to describe some of the current debates about the roles and organisation of health and welfare services in this country. There is an intensity about the debate around change and reform that can deflect care workers and managers from getting on with the work of providing services. Care workers must engage with clients and their carers to press for the right services and resources – whoever provides them. Health and welfare are highly politicised, but care workers should never forget to see issues through the perspective of the clients and the communities they serve.

This book has tried to help care workers appreciate the strengths and limitations of the main agencies involved in welfare and give some sense of how they can be made to work for people. Understanding the forces of change and the ideological push of ideas and reforms is important in developing a critical awareness of what can and cannot be done to help people.

In your own career as a helper, understanding yourself and your clients' situation is the first step in offering a sensitive caring response. It is also the basis on which you and the client can negotiate with all the systems that are and should be available to respond to clients' needs and ambitions. The notion of health and social problems is meaningless until we get some sense of how it fits in with the pattern of life of clients – what it means to them, what is at stake for them in doing something about it or leaving it, and what options for change or solutions exist. Sometimes the best we can to is to be with people, even when they don't seem to want us.

Jordan (1979) says:

'Respect for persons, as the first principle of social work, seems to me to demand that the social worker defends the rights of his clients and potential clients as if they were his own, or those of a member of his family.'

Whether you work in health or social care that seems a reasonable starting point for good care.